Responding to Human PAIN

James B. Ashbrook

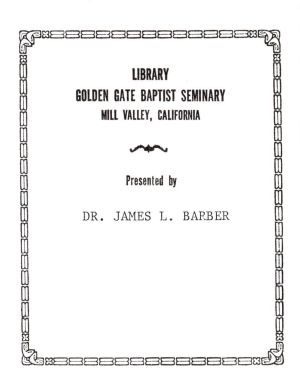
JUDSON PRESS • VALLEY FORGE

To

Responders to human pain
who through their working with me
aided my ability to respond also. . . .

Oren H. Baker
Mark Shedron
Thomas Morris
J. Lennart Cedarleaf
Frederick C. Kuether
Edward M. L. Burchard
Richard M. Johnson

RESPONDING TO HUMAN PAIN

Copyright © 1975
Judson Press, Valley Forge, PA 19481

Unless otherwise indicated, Bible quotations in this volume are in accordance with the Revised Standard Version of the Bible, copyrighted 1952 and 1971 by the Division of Christian Education of the National Council of the Churches of Christ in the United States of America, and are used by permission.

Other versions of the Bible quoted in this book are:
The Jerusalem Bible, copyright © 1966 by Darton, Longman & Todd, Ltd., and Doubleday and Company, Inc. Used by permission of the publisher.
The New English Bible. © The Delegates of the Oxford University Press and The Syndics of the Cambridge University Press 1961, 1970. Reprinted by permission.

Library of Congress Cataloging in Publication Data

Ashbrook, James B.   1925-
    Responding to human pain.

    Includes bibliographical references.
    1. Pain.   2. Suffering.   I. Title.
BJ1409.A83   253.5   75-12190
ISBN 0-8170-0677-X

Printed in the U.S.A.

Contents

Acknowledgments

The impetus for this book came from an invitation by the Clinical Theology Association of Great Britain to lead a conference at Nottingham University on "The Discipline of Counseling in Pastoral, Educational, and Social Work Settings." Frank Lake, Director, his wife and co-leader, Sylvia, the staff and tutors of the association, and the conferees afforded me a professional and personal welcome that I shall cherish always. Our time together brought forth caring and growing beyond the expectations of any of us. I am especially grateful to Marjorie Ivison for providing me with tapes of my presentations.

During the same period, the Chaplains of the Veterans Administration Hospital, Batavia, New York, under Robert F. Spencer, sponsored a lecture series by me on "Persons in Special Need." Their concerns and the response served as encouragement to share the material with a wider audience.

Material in the chapter on community resources and referrals was originally presented to an Institute on Social Welfare Services for the Clergy, sponsored by the Wisconsin State Department of Public Welfare. Their encouragement, likewise, nudged me to share the material with others.

Maxine Walaskay, with an occasional assist from Paul Walaskay, read the manuscript critically. I have a tendency to make connections in my head and assume that they are obvious to the reader when they are not. She caught as many of these obscurities as she could. The book is more readable because of her. I am grateful for her enthusiasm and encouragement.

Colgate Rochester/Bexley Hall/Crozer continues to support me in many ways. Former Dean George Brett Hall worked with my schedule so that I could accept the invitation of the Clinical Theology Association. President Leon Pacala has encouraged my ventures beyond the school for their own sake as well as for what I am able to bring back in the way of new learnings. The office staff of Mrs. Nancy Root (whose patience is magnificent) and Ms. Jackie Green, under the ever-watching and ever-prodding care of Mrs. Joanne Oliver, has enabled me to keep on when the work was difficult. Their cheerfulness in the face of my chaos constantly bolsters my morale. I have been given much by the school. I trust that my work is worthy of that support.

James B. Ashbrook

Rochester, New York

Preface

People seek help for unexpectedly varied expressions of pain.

There are hospitalized mental patients; ambulatory neurotics, often with psychosomatic complaints; those with chronic disease or disability; those in special circumstances, such as criminal offenders; those with specific stress, such as alcoholics and drug addicts; and those with sexual difficulties. The great majority of those seeking help are people whose adaptive capacities for coping get temporarily or periodically overtaxed.

Then there is the steadily increasing group that suffers from what Jerome Frank labels *weltschmerz* or world pain. "They seek help in their struggles with such problems as identity and alienation and look to psychotherapy to resolve their spiritual unrest or feelings that they are not getting all they should out of life." Their pain reflects "the confusion of moral standards and disintegration of values in today's world, as well as the increasing proportion of the educated and affluent who have the leisure and inclination to brood about such issues." [1]

The idea of "world pain," I believe, can be understood more accurately as "human pain." Of course there is physical pain. Bodily injury and biochemical disturbance can produce excruciating suffering. The same holds for animals. But I am examining the more acute *human* dimensions of pain:

> psychological pain,
>> with its locus in our sense of self and worth;
>
> sociological pain,
>> with its locus in our sense of affiliation and alienation;
>
> spiritual pain,
>> with its locus in our sense of power and meaning.

Human pain represents the personal and social and spiritual suffering people experience in the midst of living. On the levels of community and cosmos, that pain is, indeed, world pain.

While this book is intended for those who would help others professionally and/or personally, it is meant for all. Whatever specific theory and techniques of helping are described are within the concern of what it means to be human. For that reason, the book may be valuable to anyone who is reflecting on the meaning of her or his own life.

Issues raised by human pain are cognitive and experiential. We are driven to understand what is happening. In our attempts to understand, we find ourselves dealing with individual as well as universal expressions of the human pilgrimage. We look to ourselves and we look to others. Even more, we look to the universe, what it is about, how it works, what lies at its heart. Immediate concerns inevitably merge with ultimate concern.

What happens to others happens to us; what happens to us happens to others. Human pain intensifies human meaning with special poignancy. We have to make sense of that which seems senseless.

Such understanding requires our personal participation in pain. There is continuity between ourselves and others that specific stress cannot obscure. If we are to respond helpfully, we must ourselves know *of* (and not merely about) pain. In this realm we cannot be too removed from reality.

A story of Nasrudin heightens my point. Since I will be using some Nasrudin stories, let me introduce him to you here. He is a legendary Sufi character from about the third century.[2] On the surface he appears stupid. Tales about him abound. He is reported to have said, "I am upside down in this life." That parallels the description of Christians in the book of Acts (17:6) as those who have turned the world upside down. His method gradually builds up inner consciousness, shifting attention from the familiar world to true reality. Some people claim that the impact of seven Nasrudin stories, studied in succession, is enough to prepare a person for Sufic enlightenment.

One time Nasrudin caught sight of some tasty looking ducks playing in a pool. When he tried to catch them, they flew away. With that he sat down by the pool, pulled bread from his pocket, dipped the bread in the water, and started to eat. Some bystanders asked what he was doing. He replied, "I am eating duck soup."[3]

The dampness of the bread in no way compares with the delicacy of the ducks. The difference between reality and a semblance of reality is extreme. Those are, in truth, separate realities—one immediate, vivid, substantial; the other faint, insipid, spent. The residue of others' experience is inadequate for one's own sustenance. If we feed our lives on the leftovers from others' presence, the thinness of the diet makes for leanness in our soul.

How far can we usefully be from the truth?

We who would heal also need healing. We who would respond to human pain also share human pain. In his own way, when Sigmund Freud wrote an essay on "Analysis Terminable and Interminable," he was pointing to the ongoing need for the helper to be helped. For, in fact, sufferer and healer are interchanging roles: now sufferer, now healer; now helper, now helped; now giver, now receiver.

Thus, in the first section of the book, the key to "Responding" is oneself. I am in the other and the other is in me, even though in any number of specific respects we are obviously different. I use a time-limited psychotherapy case to demonstrate a process by which we can transform alienated pieces of our own experience into energizing elements for our own and others' becoming. From this critical case, I sharpen the dialectic between the polarity of receptive and active for the purpose of healing.

The remainder of the first section deals with common features in every therapeutic relationship—the ways our bodies and brains function on our behalf and the crucial demands we personally face when we venture to respond to pain. These demands complete the circle of caring, for having begun with ourselves and having reached out to others, we discover we are brought back to ourselves. If we are to care for others genuinely, we are forced to face openly who we are and what we want.

At first glance the section on "Special Pain" may appear tangential.

Dependency, aging, and dying have their own specific constellations of pain. Yet within these three experiences, the throb of human pain is present, touching each of us where we are, as we are. We come into the world; we pass through the world; we depart from the world. Our coming and our going call forth response to us from others equally with response to others from us.

Through the centuries the care of souls has tended to be individualistic. That is, the carer has seen pain on the level of individuals, separated, isolated, insulated from the settings and systems in which people live and move and have their being. The ancient claim that "there is no salvation outside the Church" reflects the deeper wisdom that sees persons within community and not by themselves. To respond caringly we must utilize the resources of the whole community. To respond effectively we must tackle outer sources of stress—in biblical language, "principalities and powers"; in behavioral jargon, systems and structures. A reviewing of what response means leads me not only to describe the availability and use of community resources, but even more to suggest a changing strategy of caring.

No matter what we do, we risk. We risk ideas and ideals, convictions and concerns, security and satisfaction. In no way can we avoid risk—either in life or in responding to pain.

In what follows I move freely between the concrete and the cosmic, between approaches to helping and meaning in life, between nuts-and-bolts and food-and-drink. I find in the core of the common the care of creation. I discover in mystery means for surviving with significance.

What we have going for us in helping and being helped is ourselves and our shared experiences. To that end, I share with you what I at present know and do in responding to my own and others' *human* pain.

THE RESPONDER

In an instant,
rise from time and space.

Set the world aside
and
become a world
within yourself.

Shabistari, *Secret Garden* [1]

1

What Is the Key: oneself

To respond . . .
To care . . .
To help . . .
To heal . . .
To reach out personally . . .
To touch pain professionally . . .
The task sounds so compelling and so attractive. One heart beats with other hearts in the presence of human pain. We are called from beyond our own little lives to enter into the lives of others.

To respond—so simple, so meaningful, so significant, so natural, so inevitable. . . .

Of course I want to respond.
Of course I want to help.
Of course I want to heal.
Of course I want to be all that I can be with others and for others and to others.

But what sounds so right and what seems so real, upon closer examination, turns into that which is unclear and uncertain. I regard the demand to be what I can be as analogous to playing a musical instrument. A story makes my point:

Nasrudin decided to play the lute. So he sought out a teacher and explored what the arrangements would be. "How much do you charge for lessons?" The teacher replied simply, "That will be ten gold pieces for the first month and one gold piece for every month thereafter."

"Excellent," exclaimed Nasrudin. "I'll begin with the second month." Or, as another version puts it, "Splendid! I shall be back in a month's time."[2]

To respond to human pain—

We can too easily jump into professional performance—or at least advanced competence—without initially paying the price of personal discipline. We want to start with the second month. That is, we want to come in when the cost is less and the burden light. We would bypass the step where the cost is greater and the burden heavier. In responding to human pain, that initial cost and that first step always mean including ourselves. To give ourselves to others in ways that matter requires that we have ourselves together as ourselves in ways that matter.

If we really intend to respond to human pain, then, of necessity, we have to start with ourselves.

Most people enter helping professions—ministry, medicine, social services, teaching, psychology—out of a personal need to be needed. At its core that need is life and health; namely, my life takes on life to the degree it is engaged with others. There can be no life without meaningful life together. But surrounding that core of human response, we find a layer of individual intent: I *will be* needed no matter what; I *will be* helpful regardless; I *will* respond at all times to all requests as requested. It is that willful drive to respond that becomes a terrible burden upon those to whom we seek to respond.

We can too easily and too casually move into responding to others' lives. We can too inadvertently and too unknowingly confuse our lives with their lives. We can too glibly and too blindly misunderstand the nature of genuine response to human pain.

Those ten gold pieces and those initial screeching notes of the first month of music lessons constitute the price and the practice of learning to play the lute of life. The one gold piece and beginning beautiful tones of succeeding months constitute the payoff and the performance of learning to play.

At the beginning, we cannot avoid looking at the personal cost and individual struggle which we must undertake if we are to put ourselves at the disposal of others. That is the necessary foundation if we are to have a self to give away in ways that matter.

What do I mean by starting with oneself?

Predicament

What we are up against as human beings can be stated simply, though it is not resolved simply. We are split—divided within and separated without. From the moment of birth, we enter into a condition characterized by distance and division.

With birth we find ourselves thrown out of the womb—out of the garden—into a confusing and confronting world. No longer are organism and environment united one with the other. Now there is a human organism and a separate world. That fundamental separation can be seen in the startle response, what psychiatrist Lawrence Kubie calls that initial gap between the organism and the environment.[3] That gap constitutes the source of all anxiety. From it all subsequent cognitive development derives.

William James emphasized the pervasive division. There is "one great splitting of the whole universe into two halves," he wrote. We make that cleavage.

> For each of us almost all of the interest attaches to one of the halves; but we all draw the line of division between them in a different place. When I say that we all call the two halves by the same names, and that those names are *'me'* and *'not me'* respectively, it will at once be seen what I mean. . . . No mind can take the same interest in [one's] neighbor's *me* as in [one's] own. The neighbor's *me* falls together with all the rest of things in one foreign mass, against which [one's] own *me* stands out in startling relief.[4]

So, we separate from the mother. Parental figures of a mother and a father grow distinguishable. Children are contrasted. Friends are identified. Male and female vary. All the divisions we discover in the outer world reflect and parallel a similar division in the inner world.

When we do not have ourselves together—when we are in many pieces—then we find ourselves constantly putting those pieces out into the world. Out there we no longer experience them as parts of us. We cease to be aware that these fragments are, in truth, expressions and extensions of ourselves. Thus they act as constant sources of difficulty and pain. As they tear at us, so we tear at others.

In contrast, you remember that in the peaceable kingdom, as Isaiah saw, the leopard and the lamb lie down together (11:6-9). Toughness and tenderness no longer tangle with each other. Your life and my life no longer limit each other. God has become all in all—the One in the many and the many in One.

So, in order for us to live with the pieces in other people's lives, it is necessary for us to begin to find our peace in the various pieces of our own lives. Only as we are somehow together—centered, integrated, whole—can we stay with the shrapnel of others.

How does one find that wholeness? What enables us to transform tearing shrapnel into tender caring? How do pieces become peace?

Possibility

The direction, I am finding, lies embedded in mystical experience as expressed in theological language. That may not be true for you, so that what I am about to explore may leave you bewildered. If that occurs, I suggest you skip ahead (to chapter 2) to my use of Gestalt therapy with a woman coping with her contemplated divorce. After that you might return to this more abstract section.

In his letter to the church at Colossae, Paul claims that the genuinely human person *is* everything and is *in* everything (1:16-17). He is referring to Jesus as the Christ, the Logos, the orderly and ordering structure of everything that is—the Word made flesh. God is not irrational will. Reality is viewed as consisting of an indwelling reasonableness and an outgoing meaningfulness. All is of a piece; nothing is apart. Change is not chaos; continuity is not constriction.

Because this language and these concepts are removed from immediate experience, I want to step back and look at them more concretely.

First, consider experiencing ourselves *as* everything. By that I mean that the basic cleavage between me and not me is overcome and undercut and wiped out. I am the world; the world is I. There is continuity between inner reality and outer reality. My internal rhythm synchronizes with the rhythm of the environment. We are a biosystem in which gradients, not boundaries, determine all form, and we live in such a biosystem.[5] All is of a piece; each is a part of the whole.

Out of the mystical tradition, Meister Eckhart provides a variety of expressions of this continuity and identification:

> So long as something is still the *object* . . . of our attention we are not yet one with the One. For where there is nothing but the One, nothing is seen.

> The Knower and the Known are one! . . . God and I, we are one in knowledge.

God is neither this nor that . . . like these manifold things. God is One.

God is the same One that I am. . . .

With Him we are one, not only as united, but in an absolute At-one-ment.[6]

In order to experience myself as everything and, therefore, as nothing, I have to be grounded in and be that which is—being itself—undifferentiated existence.[7] Our bodies provide the continuity with the world ocean of which we are a part and in which we take part. To become lost in thought and cut off from feeling is to be alienated in existence. To come to awareness by being in touch with experience is to participate in meaning. Thus our bodies, the very dwelling place of the Most High (1 Corinthians 6:19-20), provide the foundation for getting ourselves together.

The primacy of the body leads me to believe that the sensitivity movement with its emphasis on sensory awareness expresses biblical and theological understanding, namely, we get cut off from God and one another and ourselves through ignorance *and* insensitivity, lacking the ability to sense, to feel, to experience, to be as we are (Ephesians 4:18-19). And so, in sensitivity exploration people are directed to attend to their bodies and their contact with the world—around them and within them.

The process of sensory awareness results in more aliveness.[8] We are in touch and aware of our experience. For a moment we let go some of our defenses. For a moment we are open to more intense experiencing. For a moment the potentialities that lie within are more available to us. Exercises are used to shift attention from symbolic or verbal understanding to actual experience. Too often we think we feel instead of really feeling. By ignoring basic sensing, we freeze situations and ourselves, thereby anesthetizing ourselves from the richness of events.

Sensory awakening allows a rebalancing of the nonverbal aspects of the organism with the intellect. We attend to such simple bodily functions as relaxing, breathing, listening, moving, touching. This focusing helps bring us back to our senses. The process enables us to contact the source of our muscular tension. We learn how we create it. We experience the difference between tension and relaxation as we consciously and gradually let the tension go.

The way we move in sensory awareness is to listen to what our bodies are saying to us. What is outside of us is an expression of what is inside and what is inside resonates with what is outside. We heighten our sensitivity to what is on the margin, the periphery, the edges, in the shadows of our awareness rather than focus on what is out in front and clear. We are to hold up, become conscious of, what is there-and-then in order to bring it into the here-and-now.

As we make contact with that-which-has-not-been, we go on to affirm what-is-not as what-is. I am that which I experience. If my hand is twisted, as it is now, I say, "I am twisting my hand." I take responsibility. Even more, I own that which I am doing as I intensify the tension. *I* am twisting.

Once I contact what I have overlooked or denied or rejected, I again become creator-sustainer. I can create that tension and I can hold that tension. In truth, I alone create that tension and I alone maintain that tension. As I realize how I generate tension, I am on the threshold of the final step of letting that tension go by intentional relaxation. By exaggerating the muscle tension, really tightening it, I have it in hand, and by reverse intention I can allow it to cease to be. I can create that relaxation and I can maintain that relaxation. I let go and let be.

Relaxation is neither sleepiness nor droopiness. To relax means to be in "a state of aliveness," according to Bernard Gunther. We expend only the energy necessary for optimum functioning. Even in moving, excess tension is absent. We act with just the amount of effort required to accomplish the task.

Being at ease enhances what we do. Our health is better. Our learning improves. We experience more joy. To act from a base of relaxation frees us from unnecessary and excessive exhaustion. We act more effectively and more efficiently. By being at ease, our entire body operates easily; blood flows unhindered; nerves respond with alertness. We are alive and we act alive.

No function of our body is more fundamental than breathing. In and of itself, breathing presents the most direct and useful method for relaxation. When our breathing is agitated, our bodies—we—are agitated. When we hold our breath, we avoid emotion and excitement; we freeze; and we pay the price by feeling anxious. Small changes in breathing accompany amazing differences in feeling and seeing. To breathe naturally is a function of the entire organism. It is not something that we have to do; it is something that is allowed to happen. When we breathe, we are alive; when we hold our breath, we are denying life.

In Hebrew thought our souls are located in the blood stream. The Genesis portrayal of human creation emphasizes the centrality of breathing and life: and God breathed into *adam* and *adam* became a living soul (2:7). In the early period two words were used for "breath"—*ruach* and *nephesh.* Later *ruach* became synonymous with spirit or *nous* (in the Greek). It referred to that within us which related us to God. *Nephesh,* in contrast, became identified with soul or *psyche.* It designated the life principle *(vis vitalis).* For the Israelite there was no separate term for "will" as we understand it. The soul acted in its entirety through the physical organism.[9]

In the New Testament we find the differentiation of soul *(psyche)* and spirit *(pneuma)* similar to that of the later Old Testament writings. *Pneuma* (spirit) corresponds with *ruach.* They characterize the unity of power and mind as breath, i.e., "the power of life which is at the same time the bearer of the mind." Consequently, spirit is distinguished from soul but is not regarded as separate from it. For "spirit is the principle of the soul."[10] Spirit essentially involves our capacity for affinity with God. *Psyche* (soul), on the other hand, corresponds to *nephesh.* It carries primarily the Old Testament usage of "vitality" or "life" itself.

Thus, Sören Kierkegaard gave that marvelous directive to take a deep breath in faith.[11] When our breathing is constricted and shallow, we have an excess of carbon dioxide—creating anxiety—in our blood system. Then we are out of touch with where we are and who we are and what we are doing and what we want. So, with a deep breath, we recover where we are and who we are and what we are doing and what we want. No longer are we frozen or rigid. Now we are responsive and responsible.

To become aware of our breathing and to concentrate on our breathing are difficult to do. The purpose is to clear our bodies of unnecessary tensions and our minds of extraneous thoughts. We are to recover our centeredness and wholeness. Most people do not move easily from being unaware of their breathing to being aware of it. Yet the direction and process provide a bridge back from dullness to aliveness.[12]

Shift now from the idea of experiencing ourselves *as* everything to the idea of expressing ourselves *in* everything. If we are in truth "one," then we are indeed in the "many." We show ourselves in the various parts of our world. As we communicate with these parts, we converse with ourselves. There in the counterpoint of part with part we find complexity, our richness, our dynamic. No part of our world is big enough to contain all of us, yet each part of our world contains some of us. As Augustine affirmed of God, "This is not God; this is also God." Everywhere present yet nowhere contained.

In the perplexity, we find clarity. By entering into the pieces and becoming the many parts, we rediscover ourselves. Out-there-in-them we find pieces of ourselves that we have forgotten or overlooked or pushed aside. In the pieces lie the peace. By conversing with complexity, we recover our contact. In the variedness, we discover our vitality.

While we have known this in the mystical tradition, we have not, by and large, understood how to find it for ourselves. In recent years a behavioral technology has become available that can aid us in the task. Biofeedback necessitates the use of elaborate equipment; drugs require the supervision of a trained professional. Because of the risks involved and the rigor demanded, altered states of consciousness ought not to be explored casually. In contrast, one of the most helpful approaches to finding oneself in one's world has been Gestalt therapy.[13]

Gestalt is a German word meaning whole, constellation, configuration. The pattern consists of a figure which is the focal point and a ground which is the setting. The figure/ground relationship determines what is seen and what is not seen. Fritz Perls developed a therapeutic method based upon Gestalt psychology. In his approach there are several rules crucial to expressing ourselves in everything.[14] These rules assist us in recovering our several selves. When acted upon, they enable us to find in the many our one. We take back into awareness and assume responsibility for those aspects of ourselves that we have put out into the world. We recontact that which we have cut off. We reintegrate our complexity into a complementary process. As we are our projections, so we become ourselves.

There are four such rules:

1. We are to turn every other-referent pronoun—"it" or "you" or "he" or "she" or "they"—into the personal pronoun "I." Instead of using the second or third person singular or plural, we are to speak in the first person singular. Instead of saying, "My stomach is upset," say, "I 'm upset." Instead of saying, "People are always hiding what they feel," say, "I hide what I feel." The use of the pronoun "I" transforms alienated experience into owned experience.

2. We are to make the past present. We are to be here-and-now

rather than being there-and-then. What initially is not-here becomes here; what initially is not-now becomes now. In transforming lived existence into living experience, there is one qualification we need to remember. The substance, the base, the foundation, that which stands under our here-and-now, always resides out in the there-and-then. Only in eternity is there no distinction, no separation, no time, and no place. Within history there is always the complementary process of here-and-now and there-and-then. Making the past present means that the there-and-then is available to us for support and substance in our here-and-now. Being present in the past means that the here-and-now is mobilizing meaning and power in our there-and-then.

3. We are to shift from the passive mode of "having" experience to the active mode of "being" experience. Instead of reacting, we act. Instead of receiving, we initiate. Instead of waiting, we intend. We cease to be blank tablets upon whom the environment writes its script. We become writers with our own stories to tell.

4. We are to finish unfinished business. Much of the time we clutter our lives with debris from the past. A bit of it represents cherished experience; most of it constitutes crippling experience. We hang on to that which we need to let go. In theological language this "finishing" reflects the experience of grace and forgiveness. We are to push the past into the past; we are to remember to forget;[15] we are to be in the present as we live toward the future. In Gestalt therapy this requires returning in our active imagination to painful experiences that continue to haunt us. By living in them again we are able to let go of what's back there. We finish the situation. We are freed to be where we are in the here-and-now.

These Gestalt rules suggest a strategy, an approach, a method by which we can let go of the past in order to give ourselves in the present for the sake of the future.

We begin to discover a more inclusive and a more including self than we are aware of ordinarily. We become more assertive, not by "taking it out" on others, but rather by finding the courage to be as ourselves. We express more agreement, not by "giving in" to others, but rather by the courage to be part of the whole. Thus, we experience reality in our identity as human beings and express integrity in our identification with humanity as a whole.

We begin to experience the possibility of being both centered as ourselves and care-ful of others.

We begin to behave in ways that are expressive of who we are and adaptive to who others are.

The key lies within ourselves. The world ceases to be a separate and alien reality. As Meister Eckhart wrote of all creatures being one Being: "In the Kingdom of Heaven all is in all, all is one, and all is ours." [16]

2

A Case:
pieces and parts

What I have presented as the key—finding clues within oneself to what pervades one's world—has been general and abstract. While I have tied it to experiencing one's I *as* everything and *in* everything, my mystical bent has kept my point fuzzy. To overcome the difficulty, let me present excerpts from a psychotherapy case. The approach makes the point more concrete. On the basis of the case, I will describe a process which can help bring an understanding of ourselves as the key in helping and being helped.

Gestalt therapy assumes that much of our difficulty in living comes because of projection. We dissociate parts of our workaday personality and project them away from ourselves. We put upon people and things aspects of our character that we have difficulty owning.

The Gestalt technique of being our projections helps us re-own that which we have thrown out.[1] We become what we have displaced in order to be the person we are. By entering into dialogue with what we have invested out-there, we achieve a deeper and broader and more balanced integration in-here. We recover ourselves. We become who we in truth are.

Rhonda, as I shall call her, is a twenty-three-year-old nurse, married to a minister. She had contacted me two years earlier about difficulties in her marriage. At that time I saw her twice. I emphasized the importance of her sending direct messages to her husband, David, as I shall call him. Instead of passively expecting him to know what she wanted without her having to say it, she had to take initiative to let him know specifically what she wanted. Despite our limited contact, she had developed a deep and positive transference toward me. By that I mean that in me she found aspects of her relationship with her father, her brother, a sixth-grade teacher, a former lover, and her husband, all of which combined with whatever personal qualities I myself possessed.

This time she came feeling extremely anxious, neither sleeping well nor eating properly. She claimed to be on the brink of "going to pieces," vacillating between "committing suicide" and "becoming psychotic."[2]

In presenting the course of our work together, I am focusing only on conversations between pieces of herself she had projected onto others and the parts of herself she had intended as her own. I want to show how the dialogue between alienated pieces and the intended parts leads to a more integrating peace. I call this the centering-affirmation process.

In the first interview we looked briefly at her situation. She was avoiding contact with David. Her anxiety level was high. She saw as alternatives separating or becoming trapped in a meaningless marriage. She had high expectations of me. I was her only hope. Much of her drive for love from older men came, as she indicated, from searching for a father to take care of her as a little child. I ended the session emphasizing that our time would be limited to the academic semester. I indicated that we would work on reducing the gap between the little girl and the woman's body. We would seek to find what she wanted that was appropriate, while looking at, living with, and giving up the inappropriate.

The Shock of Recognition

The initial movement of centering-affirmation takes place in what I call the shock of recognition. In the pieces, one must see one's own presence. To discover the truth of one's self is startling.

The task requires clarifying what one-in-one's-several-pieces wants. That takes time. What one feels one wants seldom turns out to be what one *truly* wants. To arrive at genuine wants, one must contact what one has expressed indirectly through one's projected pieces. In Rhonda's therapy this initial movement of recognition came in a dominant projected pattern, culminating in a preliminary centering of her supposed wants.

A Little Girl and a Grown Woman

By the second session ambivalence about her marriage had surfaced. She wanted to leave, yet was afraid to leave. She characterized her marriage as "blah." She had manipulated her husband into taking care of her. Her pattern was to get others to be responsible. That way she could blame others—in this instance David—for whatever happened.

"What is it that *you* want, Rhonda?"

Her answer begins to sharpen one side of her inner split. "As a little girl, I want to be taken care of."

I ask her, "Can you talk to me as a little girl?"

Quickly and easily she is a little girl three years old. *"I want somebody to comfort me when I hurt, to be happy with me when I'm happy, uh, to be there, to take responsibility for me."* She pauses and then continues more thoughtfully. *"To know that somebody is there because I'm afraid of myself, you know. I'm not sure that I am enough by myself."*

With that insight she returns to her present conflict. "I think that's part of the huge hang-up about leaving David, you know; at least David is somebody."

With her beginning to make contact with the one side, I ask her to contact that other side. "Now talk to me as a woman."

She responds with the confidence of a twenty-eight-year-old.

"I want to be able to give, uh, in many ways—physically, intellectually, sexually. I want to be admired and respected, you know, both as a person and as a professional. I want to share with someone important to me, you know. I don't just want to give. I want to share."

More rapidly, now, I shift her psychic center back and forth between grown woman and little girl.

"Talk to me as a little girl."

"I want people to give to me. I want people to love me and hold me and tell me that everything is going to be all right."

"Talk to me as a woman."

"I want to be able to make a decision and take the consequences for whatever I decide. I want to be able to recognize that in life right and wrong just are not clear-cut, you know, as far as a lot of decisions you have to make. There isn't any right or wrong. You take the consequences of whichever way you take and don't worry about black and white. I want to do satisfying things, things that I get satisfaction from."

With the emergence of satisfying strength, I ask her to respond as her own centered self. "Now talk to me as Rhonda, standing between the little girl and the grown woman."

"I think I want to be able to stand on my own two feet because the fleeting whim says that I've had [love and care]. It's a really powerful feeling, but I'm really, really scared. I want people to love me and I want to love back, but I'm not sure I know how to love back."

She was right about not knowing how to love maturely; yet at the moment I wanted to focus on her developing strength and the underlying fear.

"What could happen if you stood on your feet?"

"Falling over and not being able to get up. What I'd want is for somebody to come and pick me up, but probably, you know, I would pick myself up again. It wouldn't be a total disaster."

The little girl part of her wanted me to make her decision about staying or leaving. The rational woman part did not.

Much of the next interview dealt with her anger at me, her supervisor, her former lover, her husband. She became self-conscious toward the end, wondering what I saw when I looked at her.

Stiffness, flatness, a hint of bubbliness, potentially "a lovely lady."

"That's wonderful to hear. That . . . I don't have to be stiff, cold, unhappy and that you care enough to help me out."

A Seductive Young Woman

In the waiting room the next week, Rhonda felt "awkward" for the first time. It consciously "hit" her that she was a client.

David had visited his parents. During the visit he had tried to interpret to them the pending separation. He told them about Rhonda's seeing me and of her problem of relating to me as part of her pattern of seeking a father figure. Rhonda was furious.

During the four days of his absence, she attempted to discover what it would be like to be on her own. She visited a friend who lived in "hippie town." She reveled in the fun of knowing she could stay out as late as she wanted and "not have anybody to worry about." No longer did she need David to meet her dependency needs.

That supposed autonomy, however, proved deceptive. She was using a lot of other people as "substitute" dependency objects. She connected her "crush" on me as part of the pattern—first her sixth-grade teacher; currently a colleague in a seminar on group work; most acutely, her defense against involved fantasies with me. She sought closeness, yet feared it.

This day Rhonda had appeared strikingly attired in a low-cut dress. She commented on it.

"I've thought a lot about last time and being cold and not wanting to be that way." She pauses before becoming explicit. "I did something different today. I wore this dress, which is a miracle, because I bought this dress about two months ago and haven't had nerve enough to wear it. I thought my hesitation might have been because my supervisor (a woman) had commented to me one time that I always wore high necklines. And so I did it," she laughingly suggests, "as acting-out. You know, 'I'll show you I can wear the lowest neckline I can find. . . .'"

Now, she feels, she is not wearing it to act-out. Instead she is wearing it "mainly . . . you know, because at least I'm trying not to be uptight."

"A little more open," I interpret, "a little more loose. More of yourself showing."

"Yeah," she agrees readily. "And it's not particularly uncomfortable."

Just prior to starting our therapeutic work, Rhonda had dreamt of walking down a city street in flannel pajamas unbottoned at the top, looking for her sixth-grade teacher. Now, she exclaims, "I can reveal myself without unbuttoning my pajamas or without having my pajamas unbuttoned. . . . It's kind of fun in a way, too. . . . I feel like I'm attractive. Flannel pajamas aren't attractive at all." She feels less like the tomboy, as in the past, and more like a woman—a young woman. "I'm feeling like maybe I've moved from nine to eighteen."

We move into the area of what she wants, as an eighteen-year-old, from me. She begins to allow her thoughts to wander. *"I think at first I would fantasize doing things with you . . . like taking walks . . . maybe of even going to the zoo."* Her self-above-self intrudes. "That's kind of like a five- or six-year-old."

She continues," . . . *going to a play or something that we both would enjoy. Uh, sitting in front of the fireplace having a nice conversation, not an office-type conversation. . . . I think having you hold me, only not in a little girl sense. . . . We are sitting by the fireplace. . . . And I'm very soft and pretty and appealing to you and you are very appealing to me . . . and instead of you holding me, you might lay your head in my lap . . . and I'm wanting for us to make love."* With that she consciously stops her fantasizing.

She wonders what I am thinking of her fantasy. Behind her wonder lurks the question of what I am thinking of her. I experience her on the verge of crying. "Maybe," she muses, "feeling like I'll get lost in my fantasies and wanting to know how to relate them to reality."

With that, I use the closeness and the questioning to instruct her nascent self.

"For the child, the reality and the fantasy are virtually the same. For the adult there is a difference between fantasy and reality. The six-year-old in you experiences the fantasy as close to reality."

Rhonda is responding with "mmhmms" and "yeahs." Her nodding head and facial expression convey to me the clarifying process getting through.

"Fantasies," I continue, "reflect the reaching and longing inside of us which we cannot utilize for our own growth until we take them into ourselves and allow them to take us where they will in our fantasy. But that isn't reality. It's the source out of which solid reality comes. As long as you back off from your fantasies taking you there, you aren't going to assimilate all this stuff that's going on inside you."

As I try to stand under her freer experiencing, I also set up limits.

"There is probably as little likelihood of our going to a play together or sitting in front of a fireplace as making love or going to a zoo." Her "mmhmms" continue. "But if I turn that off, it does reflect the distancing, the apprehension, about the closeness. And I suppose the fact that you don't fully accept what you experience yourself, as well as being afraid of what I think about you, keeps you both too young and too old."

I pause and then summarize in a way to encourage her growing sense of self. "I am pressing you to move into your fantasies because your inner life is not regressive, childish, chaotic, destructive. Your inner life is growing a beautiful and adaptive and constructive self."

Having moved into the dependency of her little girl and the desirable grown woman self, Rhonda had begun to incorporate and coordinate these several selves. The result came forth as a venturesome and somewhat seductive younger woman. As such, she wanted to translate fearful fantasies into fulfilled realities. The vitality of her cut-off and alienated parts had begun to flow. As she could allow herself to "be" the little girl *and* the desirable grown woman, she could begin to come together as herself. Much work remained to be done, but the forces for centering-affirmation were moving.

The Confrontation of Intentions

The middle movement of centering-affirmation comes with what I call the confrontation of intentions. In the parts, one must assert one's presence consciously and deliberately.

The task requires escalating confrontation between the several selves. It is painful. What one *thinks* one fears seldom turns out to be what one *genuinely* dreads. But to arrive at real dread—the dizziness of possibility—one must aggressively claim what one intends indirectly through the pieces as well as directly through the parts.

In Rhonda's therapy this middle movement of challenging intentions developed through three projected patterns, culminating in a sharpened split of her supposed possibilities.

Angry Wife and Angry Husband

With acknowledgment of the distance between them, Rhonda and David both began acting assertively. She used work and school as reasons for not being home. In retaliation he labeled her behavior "bad" and "selfish." She pressured him to go to a marriage counselor as a way to take the pressure off of her and put it back on him.

While Rhonda's behavior suggested her desire to separate, her attitude revealed fright. The prospect of escalating anger terrified her. She imagined David would either strangle her or stab her. More exploration brought us to her own unexpressed anger.

"I might kill somebody, too," she acknowledged. "My fantasies to get out of the marriage were always that David was going to die. Not that I was going to kill him, but I've been killing him in my fantasies for a long time. . . ."

If she really let her emotions out, she felt she would stab him to death. A fragment from the past burst into consciousness. "What's coming to me right now is that I can remember being just fantastically angry with my brother as children and fighting and biting and clawing and squeezing and kicking." Rather than killing David with a knife, she saw the scratching and tearing of children scrapping. She wanted to blow up at him yet feared his blowing up in retaliation. "I'd like to get rid of some of my anger, but, uh, I'd have to take his in return."

Again we were presented with an opportunity to sharpen the isolated parts of her working personality.

"Suppose we invite David to come in and sit in this chair." We imagine he has joined us. "What is it you want to say to him?"

"I'm angry as hell at you because you sit there like a passive blob and won't do anything. You make me feel guilty for everything I try to do and . . . you don't give a damn about me most of the time. Or at least you don't show me that you do. And you. . . ."

"Now go and be David."

"I think what you did with Donald [the man she had had an affair with] was the rottenest thing that anybody has ever done. Nice married people don't have affairs with people when they are engaged and they don't run around loving their therapists [like she 'loved' me], and I think you're a dirty, immoral person and you want to run out and play with your girl friends and I don't want you to because you should stay home and cook and clean for me, and I'm tired of you always wanting to do all your own things. . . ." And so her anger and hurt and resentment and guilt pour out.

I signal for her to become her conscious intended self.

"Go to hell!" She snaps back at her lost piece. "I can't help what happened and I've got to be me for a while and I do cook and clean. So there, what are you bitching about?"

"Now be David."

"Yes, but you never stay home and you never want to be interested in the things I'm interested in. And besides that, I don't trust you. I think you are going to run around and seduce men behind my back." The tone comes through more moderately, more longingly, more fearfully. *"Besides,"* he-she continues, *"I don't know why I ought to change."*

"If you want to stay married to me," assertive Rhonda declares, "you are going to have to change, because I don't like you the way you are. I don't like what you are doing to me. I don't like the way you are reacting to the way I've changed. And besides that, you are trying to make me a captive. You are trying to do what my father did to my mother. You're trying to tie me to you and your profession and to

your children that I don't want to have and to your house and to your
stupid church. . . ."

She moves into a long, pensive silence.

"Now be David."

*"Yeah, but you knew about my house and about my stupid church
and my children all before you married me. So why the hell did you
marry me?"*

"I don't know why I married you. Because I don't even like you
very much right now. When I married you, I didn't know anything
about love and I had no idea who I was or what I wanted to be. And
I'm mad as hell at myself for marrying you."

The exchange ended. The sides had been expressed. Her centered
self had begun to see her lost self in the several parts.

"OK," I shift her awareness from experiencing to reflecting. "Now
what's happened? What have you experienced?"

She pauses. "Seeing David's side some. A kind of overwhelming
sense of responsibility. I really did know all this stuff when I married
David. . . . And I think maybe I married him for kicks and nothing
else and feel very responsible now that it's not kicks any more and
that, uh," she pauses mobilizing more of her latent strength to take
the next step, "that I'm going to have to be the one who gets out of the
marriage if I want out and that if I stay in, I've got to accept the
responsibilities." She pauses again and then, almost sheepishly, softly
adds, "I also felt good to be talking with David."

Reality demanded responsibility. Responsibility meant "playing it
straight." At the moment it seemed more appealing to play it straight
and leave than to play it straight and stay. Feelings of sadness and
responsibility enveloped her.

"I am trying to sort out what playing it straight with David would
really mean. And I guess what I am seeing is that part of what it
involves is going along with taking the responsibility and showing
him that I'm desperately sad and sorry for what I've done. . . . And
that hurts. . . ."

An Active Part and an Entangled Piece

Rhonda and David talked after that. The confrontation did not
turn out to be as "bad" as she had feared. He intended to do his own
therapeutic work; she had to intend to do hers.

Now the time-limited nature of our contract sharpened her fear of
being deserted. On the one hand, she felt that I was simply "using" her

for my own teaching purposes, without caring for her. On the other, she dreamed that I loved only her; she was all I had. Several times she allowed herself, for the first time, to daydream of our making love, which left her feeling frightened. Concurrently, feelings of my having deserted her two years previously reappeared.

"I still feel like I'm hung up somewhere," she informs me. "That I'm still not really able to let you see me, you know. I'm saying it hurts and feeling like I'm going to cry but like I still feel there's a wall."

"Can you tell me what the wall is for?"

"It's like . . . it's in me. There's still something very uptight and very tense."

"Can you close your eyes for me. See the wall. Describe it. Tell me what you are doing in relation to it."

"It's a great big tall brick wall. It's got barbed wire at the top. It's a fairly flat surface so that it's hard to climb. And I never was really very good at climbing. Somewhere I'm running, trying to find a way to go around it instead of over it. And the ends of it are very, very far away, but I think they are there."

"But they are out of sight?"

"Right now, yeah." Instead of resorting to her passive stance she responds more actively. *"So I'd like to try and find things that I can stack up so that I can get over. But there isn't anything there. And there is that barbed wire at the top."* She pauses, contemplating available resources. *"What I am going to do is take off at a dead run for one of the ends of the wall . . . but it's kind of like it's just out of reach. . . . Just a little bit farther than I can go."*

"Well, why don't you get acquainted with the wall?" I suggest, firmly believing that in the center of the obstacle lies the blessing.

"It's a red brick wall."

"Can you feel it?"

"Yeah. It's rough."

"Are you just touching it lightly or are you really feeling it?"

"I'm rubbing my hand all over it. It's going to take the skin off my fingers if I do it any harder."

"OK."

"And it feels like it's strong. It doesn't feel like I could knock it down. But I'd like to try to knock it down and kick it. But when I kick it, it hurts my foot. I feel like if I were a little bigger maybe I could push it over. The top of it is three or four feet out of my reach. But if I got to the top, I'd be in the barbed wire." She pauses. *"It would hurt to*

be in the barbed wire, but I really want to know what's on the other side. But what I'm afraid of is that I am going to just sit there and do nothing."

"OK." I simply try to encourage her to stay with what is.

"I'm getting frustrated now because I feel like I really can't get over that wall. . . . Only I'm not trying hard enough or I'm trying the wrong way." More silence. *"There isn't anybody else around, but there are a lot of trees."* More silence. *"They are not close enough to the wall."* More silence. *"I'm jumping up and down to try to grab the top of the wall now. . . ."*

"So you need to grow some." I turn physical features of the fantasy into their psychic counterparts.

"I'm getting more and more frustrated." More silence and more silence and more silence. *"I don't know what to do."* More silence. *"I'm still trying to jump to get over it."*

"Can you explore the wall some more?"

"The plaster in there is kind of old and crumbly."

"Crumbly?"

"When you rub it hard with your fingers, it comes out. The bricks look like the bricks—in fact, the whole wall looks like the wall that was around the backyard of my house when I was a little girl. The bricks are that color—kind of a dark purplish-red. If I had a sledgehammer, I could knock the wall down. It's kind of a pretty wall except for the barbed wire."

What a mixture of barrier and possibility, of present and past, of helplessness and assertiveness, of decay and delight.

"Then the wall's not all bad."

"It keeps me from knowing what's on the other side. And the other side looks nicer. It's got nice green grass and the trees are nicer and there are people on the other side." She pauses and then continues. *"If I had wings, I could fly to the other side, but the wall is out of place."*

A sudden transition intrudes.

"I just jumped out of a tree and onto the top of the wall. I'm getting stuck by the barbed wire. I'm getting all tangled up in it and it's hurting. It's sticking me in lots of different places and it's hard to get untangled. I have to do it slowly, very slowly, so I don't get hurt."

"There's no rush," I counsel, even though the future feels like it is collapsing in upon her.

"Yes there is because I am in a hurry to get to the other side."

As she became entangled in the barbed wire, she felt like somebody was stabbing her on her chest. She grew consciously anxious. The issue had ceased to be a wall between herself and where she wanted to get and had become, instead, the fact that in order to get untangled she would have to risk more hurt.

"Anything I do now is going to hurt. If I just sit here and let the wall stay, I'm going to wind up still hurting and yet I might crash through the wall and it's still going to hurt me."

Out of her confusion Rhonda asked me to hold her hand.

"And what would holding my hand mean?"

"That I was touching you and letting you touch me, sort of like breaking the wall."

Panic and Possibility

A "wild week" followed. Great ups and tremendous downs.

One way to start getting out of the barbed wire, she had decided, was finding a job. An ideal possibility opened—something concrete that helped focus the other side of the wall. The future did not loom as "a total blank."

Then she and David talked in more detail about her leaving. The accumulation of "little reasons" appeared to add up to separation. With that Rhonda had started to panic. She had cried and cried and cried, sobbing and sobbing and sobbing. "But then what happened really scared me because I started in just vomiting violently; I vomited like ten or twelve times."

In part she saw the vomiting as a move to get David to be nice to her and thus avoid talking anymore about her leaving. She suspected that he wanted her to leave more than she wanted to leave. Surprisingly to her, they laughed together and enjoyed each other the following two days as they had not in a long time. Then in the session, she began experiencing a similar helplessness.

"I'm torn between thinking, yeah, I really can cope with it and, you know, I can't; I'm lost; I'm sunk."

"So inside," I interpret, "you experience—what—a great gap between the panic and the possibility?"

"Yeah." I had been on target. "Between the part of me that's just immobilized and not functioning at all and the part of me that is, you know, really functioning lots better than I was. You know, I'm feeling the gap just widening out."

Instead of coming together, her several parts were pulling her apart.

"Well, let's try getting these parts to talk. Let's put the Possibility over here (in this empty chair) and the Panic over here (in this other chair)."

"I'll do Panic first." By now she had learned how to move into the pieces more easily. *"Uh, I can't reach you, Possibility, because I'm too scared and because I'm not just me in this alone. . . ."*

"You aren't very convincing," I contend.

She accepts my feedback while stressing the difficulty of the task.

"I've never had to do this before. Nobody's ever said, 'Make this kind of decision. You have to really decide. You can't go on having fun forever. You have to decide something's really important.' That's going to be hard to back out of and face the fact that, uh, maybe David doesn't really love me. Uh, and that's an awful way to feel. It's very confusing and I don't know where I'm going." Her identification with Panic comes through more persuasively. *"I have just a complete, horrible desire to give up. I have to do something and I'd rather just totally, completely give up."*

From across the room she answers as Possibility.

"But look. You haven't given up already because you've, uh, done lots of constructive things at the present. And you've given yourself a future. And you know you can cope. So you are being stupid and silly. And if David doesn't really love you, then you've just got to face that, because maybe that's just the way things are, and maybe somebody else will love you. You aren't totally unlovable. You are functioning beautifully at work. You are doing well in school. Your professor wants to give you a job. In fact, she was delighted to give you a job. It's a good job and a job you can do and it's an exciting job. . . ."

Now Panic has her comeback.

"Yeah, but that's a year away and I've got to move now. I've got to do something now. I've got to face my family in terms of my grandmother's thinking that people who get divorced are awful and of all of the pressure she is putting on us. I've got to face that I've got to move if I leave. If I don't leave, I've got to really try, which I'm not sure I want to do. I've got to go out to dinner with all of those people in the church. I've got to try to get excited about David's work, which I'm not sure I can do, but I'm not sure I can move either. . . ."

Panic pauses. Weakly she protests, *"Always before, somebody else has decided for me, and nobody is doing that this time."*

Possibility picks up the conversation.

"You are handling it better than you ever have. Besides that, your family is thousands of miles away and you don't have to put up with them very often anyway. So you are an adult now. You can make decisions. You've made some decisions before. . . . So it's not really all that scary. You've got to shape up and be an adult. And besides that, you can do it."

After that moral bracer I ask her to return to her self-above-selves. "And what would Rhonda say of these two people? What do you think," I wonder, "observing their interaction?"

"That it is still kind of a helpless crybaby over there—mad as hell at the world because it is not going to make a decision for her. Uh, coming up with . . . not very good reasons for not being able to make a decision, but scared."

"So," I sharpen, "the panic is real but the reasoning is phony."

"Yeah, yeah. Which I think is part of what's confusing about it, because the reasons I can put my finger on for the panic just aren't that good."

"And what about the possibility part?"

"This person is becoming much more me, uh, in terms of getting more comfortable with doing adult sorts of things and being, you know, more capable and willing to take more kinds of responsibility. And, I think, being able to look at things more realistically."

To choose to stay meant she would have to be more active in David's work. The prospect evoked resentment. Behind that lurked the question of whether she wanted to be bothered about anyone. What she was experiencing felt "adolescent."

"I adolescently rebelled by getting married at nineteen, and now at twenty-three I've got to rebel adolescently by getting unmarried."

Rhonda left the session feeling the strength needed for the decision. She also left "much more alive."

A Child at the Zoo and an Adult at a Museum

In the week that followed, the conflict climaxed. We had been saying some "terribly, terribly painful" things. She did not like looking at them, but knew she had to. Then a mistake with a patient of hers at work and a misunderstanding with her advisor combined to sharpen internal pressure. The bottom seemed to drop out.

Rhonda described what had happened: "I was all curled up in a fetal position and I was just, you know, well, I scared the dog. The dog started barking and, uh, and I remember having the thought, 'You aren't a baby. You're more like an animal.' It was further down than being a baby, which was really scary."

She had been obsessed about wanting to telephone me, and finally had. Through the experience she began to see that she had wanted more from me and from her husband than either of us could give. Even so, "the baby side" of her kept intruding and demanding. She thought that "maybe one of the reasons that the little girl is still there is that, uh, I know this sounds dumb," she acknowledges, "but I think I grew up too soon." She had always been told to "grow up. You can't act like that." So part of her felt like "I've always been very, very old."

Once again the split within her centered self allowed us to explore her becoming the piece and the part.

"What would you do if you were very, very young?" I ask.

Rhonda hesitates and then quickly responds, *"Daddy would take me to the zoo. And it would be all right to get mad and cry sometimes because I was a child and children do that. . . ."*

After contacting the past, I bring her into the present. "And what would you do now if you were very, very little?"

"I'd do happy things. I'd have Mommy and Daddy read stories to me and, uh, be there when I wanted them."

"Which would be when?"

"On the weekends when they always sent us to stay with our grandparents and I never wanted to go. I'd get to stay home. And I'd have them, you know. They'd be interested in what I was doing. I'd have a father who knew the names of my friends." Little Rhonda pauses.

Big Rhonda intrudes. "But, you know, I think my feeling is that that's never going to happen. I need to learn how to get satisfaction out of being an adult, which, in some ways, I've started to do—some of the things we talked about last week. I'd better grow up and know how to be married."

In fact, she and David had begun to share some satisfying activities, such as going to an art museum. They found they could "just enjoy being with each other and that was good enough." I sought to clarify the contrast.

"What's the difference between going to an art museum with David and going to the zoo with Daddy?"

In terms of "doing," not much. In terms of meaning, considerable. "Going to the art museum with David, we'd be on the same level. . . . I have something to give as well as something to take. We could have fun, kind of as equals. Uh, you know, I think going to the zoo with Daddy would be kind of being catered to, which as a very little girl would have been nice but, you know, part of me is not a little girl and that part likes to be equal."

That, however, did not add up to enough to remain married. They had talked about her rejection of the church and his anger over her lack of interest. No longer was he content to let her indecisively drift in their relationship. He demanded a decision.

Rhonda's expectation took on a more realistic shape. The relationship demanded emotional investment. Yet, she admits, "I am beginning to see that I can still be invested in David and not totally lose my identity, because I think my identity is getting stronger. Before, I think I was feeling like 'if I invested, I was going to get swallowed up.' I've seen the possibility now that I can be married to David and still be me."

She still found reasons to postpone telling him that she had decided to stay. In talking with a friend about therapy, her "love" for me accentuated her "sadness" at having to grow up and stop being a little girl.

The transforming process inevitably takes the form of a responsive centering. Because one is including one's several selves, the task of testing out recognized intentions proves exhilarating. What one *knows* one chooses usually turns out to be what in truth one wanted. When this realization comes, the dizziness of possibility changes into the excitement of discovery.

In Rhonda's therapy this climaxing movement of recognizing *her* intentions disclosed itself through various responsible relationships and activities, culminating in an appropriate termination of the therapeutic contract.

Having asserted her "rights" as an angry wife *and* having condemned her actions as "irresponsible" as an angry husband, Rhonda found herself painfully entangled. Her involvements in the here-and-now, isolated from her there-and-then, cut off possibilities on the other side of her separate selves. As such possibilities came closer, her panic mounted. The result crystallized in the alternative of either becoming a child, catered to by a male-father figure, or becoming an adult, sharing with a male companion. She saw and set the directions in which she could choose to invest her self-above-selves.

Recognition of Choices

The transforming movement of centering-affirmation appears with what I call the recognition of genuine choices. A person combines the vital self in the pieces with the intended self of the parts. One becomes more truly *one.*

An Adult Relationship

The next day Rhonda wrote me a letter. For the first time the "watchers" behind the mirror had disturbed her. (Some of the center staff had been observing the therapy as part of their training.) She hoped by writing that I could help her have "the courage" to deal with her feelings "face-to-face, in spite of our 'audience.'" She could not make a decision about David until she had discussed how she felt about me and, by inference, how I felt about her.

Rhonda entered the session confused. She had taken my refusal to take responsibility for her staying or leaving as an encouragement to leave. More than that, she thought that if she left I would divorce my wife and marry her. She had confused my feeling of responsiveness at what I saw as her blossoming life with her hope for love from me.

Once clear about our relationship, she proceeded to explore the work required to find grown-up satisfactions in her marriage. She and David had agreed to take professional leadership in a program they could do together. She realized, with amusement, that "it's much easier being in love with somebody you're not married to, because you don't have to turn his undershirts back the right way."

From having wanted to be a little girl taken care of by me as a kindly father, she had come to feel she could give to me as a grown-up. Then she reported, "I'm just sitting here and getting less scared about loving you; still loving you but not being as scared about it and feeling, beginning to feel like, you know, I'm probably going to still love you when I walk out of here in May, but that's all right. Maybe in a way that's the big step because with [Donald] I always had the feeling that it wasn't all right to love him."

Some Reality Testing

During this period Rhonda had attended a professional conference. She went with conflicting feelings and returned ecstatic. It had loomed as a "scary" test of trying out her "new me." To her amazement she discovered that she "really had something to offer people—my enthusiasm, my openness, my willingness to learn, plus some real intelligence that I was willing to put to work in a new situation."

She also made "decisions"—nothing earth-shattering, but simple and real. "Whether or not to go to a party when I felt I needed to study—but before it would have been hard for me to decide. The ambivalence was still there—I still needed to study—to stay in the room alone and study with no big regrets."

Temporary Flight into Regression

This next session marked the only time she arrived late for our appointments. The first part consisted of Rhonda's spilling over about the conference. She had acted in ways that had enabled her to shape it rather than let it shape her. The change from a passive object into an active subject was decisive.

Along with her excitement, I sensed underlying anxiety. I wondered what it meant.

She talked of obvious stresses and then paused. "It was funny because yesterday I was kind of afraid I wasn't going to want to come today. But I did," she hastily added, "when I got up this morning."

We began exploring the shadowy nuances. She discovered she wanted to leave me before I "left" her with our termination. At the same time she is "feeling very much like a helpless baby right now," wanting to curl up with my arms around her. She feels we have not dealt with something that is big and basic, yet she is unable to identify what it might be.

That day had been a flight into regression. It marked the remaining resistance to the pending termination. It equally marked the more adult relationship growing between us.

Limiting and Loving and Leaving

Like the Watergate concertos, just when developments get crucial the tape gets jammed. Trouble developed with the sound equipment during the next two sessions. Understandably, the observers found it frustrating to watch yet hear nothing. In a strangely providential way, one of the women staff members had left and then returned the second week. She wondered if she could pick up anything nonverbally. And she did!

Toward the end of that session, Rhonda and I had moved from our regular seating arrangement. I had sat in the big easy chair. She had curled up on the floor at my feet. Together we had shared our own private fantasy of sitting quietly before a crackling fire in a snowbound cabin in the woods. It had been peaceful and beautiful. When the hour was up, wc had kissed—tenderly and lovingly.

The following week Rhonda and I met with those who had been observing us through the months.

Rhonda referred immediately to our previous session. "I think when we started, if anything would have bothered me, it would have been people watching last week. But it didn't bother me at all. I really felt good, like, 'You would have missed the best part if you had missed last week.'"

After several spoke of their appreciation and awe and learning from her therapy, the woman who had seen but not heard us told of her own feelings. "I'm really not sure how to describe [what I saw] other than that it was to me quite an emotional experience. The most interesting thing to me was that I picked up what I thought was a fireside."

Others did not yet know what had happened.

"It was Jim and Rhonda," she clarified. "They had moved over to the large chair on this side of the room. And Jim was sitting in the chair and Rhonda was sitting on the floor next to him."

"What preceded that," I explained, "was that after about twenty minutes I told Rhonda I was feeling very distant; that we were quite far apart; that what I had imagined in my mind was her coming over and sitting down on the floor by me, which, I guess," I turned to the staff woman, "you had been feeling, too."

"I felt the distance between the two of you." She agreed.

"So, then," I went on to explain, "instead of coming over to where I was sitting, Rhonda moved over to the big chair, the more comfortable chair. So that's where we were then."

"And I picked up the feeling," the woman continued, "that it was more like a fireside. It was very hard to say that afterwards to Jim because, you know, I thought, 'There's no fireplace in here.'" Everyone laughed uproariously as we shared a fantasy world together. "But that was the feeling that I had. And afterwards Jim had said that you, Rhonda, had mentioned something about a fireplace a long time ago."

"Yeah," Rhonda chimed in. "My comment was that it reminded me of the fantasy I had had about sitting by a fireplace."

"It was a very warm feeling," the woman acknowledged.

Rhonda returned to her fantasy fears. "I think it was especially meaningful to me, too, in terms of being able to break down the fear that I've had of relationships with older men. That, uh, the same thing that happened with [Donald] was going to keep repeating. It was going to be a pattern. And last week I really finally realized that I had self-control with it. And that sort of thing wasn't going to happen over and over again. But that, you know, I could still have warm, close, enjoyable kinds of relationships and not get carried away and feel guilty about it."

Our conversation turned to the dramatic changes which had taken place in Rhonda. Initially, she had come across as such an uninteresting person, a little child, an emotional drag, a flat person. Lately, she had come through as so alive.

Then the time-limited nature of the contract came to the fore.

"I'm not sure I would have changed," Rhonda surprised us all by saying, "or I would have been very frightened of changing if I had realized that as soon as I had changed and grown up, then, you know, I would have had to terminate. I think I would have had a much more difficult time going through the process of change knowing that I was going to lose you [Jim] as soon as I changed. So that by knowing there was a time limit, I think I made a lot more progress than I would have."

"So there was no punishment, then, for getting better?"

"Yeah."

After meeting with our observers, Rhonda and I held a shortened session. She focused exclusively on what our relationship would and could become. It could *not* be like that with her sixth-grade teacher. She did *not* want it to be one-sided anymore, with my doing all the giving and her doing all the getting. She explored ways by which our relationship might become that of colleagues. Definitely, in the event of "big trouble," I would be the person she would contact. In "times of great happiness" she might contact me also.

For our last time together we chose not to be observed.

Rhonda spoke of "feeling very sad and hurting and yet feeling good at the same time." She had met pressure deadlines. Instead of experiencing "a big letdown," she had "started thinking about what an incredible semester it had been. How many things have changed. I've got a really good possibility of pulling A's in my two courses, which just absolutely amazes me," she informed me. Then she summarized, "You know, I was thinking, 'Gee, I've changed my life.

I've made my marriage work.' And lots and lots of things."

She spoke of fantasizing about David and her bringing their first-born child to see me whenever it arrived. "And part of that fantasy," she added, "was sitting in your office, breast-feeding the baby which, you know, when I thought about that, I thought, 'Wow, that's loaded!' And yet the more I thought about it, the more I thought in lots and lots of ways it shows how far I've come."

"How do you mean?" I wonder. Even to the end I want to avoid doing her work for her. Even to the end I want her to be explicit in what she says to me and not to assume I know what is in her mind without her having to say.

"In that, you know, when I first came to see you, I couldn't give. I just wanted to get from you. And the fantasy was very much of coming to your office and being able to give to a child. In January I was absolutely petrified at the thought of motherhood, which doesn't scare me anymore. I don't want to get pregnant right away because there are other things I want to do, but it wouldn't be the absolute end of the world if I did. And, you know, just the whole thing was—I went to sleep after that, and when I woke up I felt just really nice and warm and good."

The warmth of closeness and the sadness of separation are very much in the foreground of our relationship at this moment.

"I feel like I want to hug you," she ventures. It is a direct request, much different from her sitting passively and indirectly wanting responses.

"One of the things that's the very most important to me," she picks up after we have hugged each other, "is that I can love you very, very much and be very attracted to you and not have to get frightened of it. I can like it and enjoy it for being something very good."

She goes on to speak of trust and openness.

"How does trust come in?" I wonder.

"I guess, in part, knowing that, uh, we're not going to do anything that's going to make either of us guilty. What that day [when we fantasized being in front of the fireplace] meant to me was that I could be attractive without being irresistible."

"You're not going to lose control, nor do you have to maintain control."

A bit later, to continue finishing the situation, I ask her how she decided on the dress she is wearing.

"It's new, so it was something I hadn't worn before. I like it. David brought it to me from his last trip. I think I look pretty in it."

"So it really kind of picks up a whole bunch of things." I am pleased with the multidimensional symbol. "It's the newness. David got it for you while he was away. And you do look pretty in it. Not seductive but attractive."

From tying up the past, I turn our attention to the future. What are her plans? What are her projects? What is she working on? She, in turn, asks about what I will be doing.

And so ends our contract!

Follow-up

I want to add a follow-up.

We did, in fact, bump into each other occasionally in the course of our various activities. The meetings were brief, casual, comfortable. Then, one day two years later I received a phone call. She wanted to come to see me. She had "a surprise."

The surprise was a healthy baby boy! While she did not breast-feed the youngster in front of me, she did share her excitement with motherhood.

A year later she came to say "good-bye." They were moving from the area because David was assuming the pastorate of another church. Their baby was developing rapidly. They were continuing to grow in their marriage. She was arranging to work part-time.

Another year passed. In a Christmas note Rhonda wrote: "We were happy to learn that I'm expecting again. I am really enjoying parenthood. I'm not planning to look for work again until after the baby comes. . . . Christmas finds us all well and happy."

And so her life goes on. From having been her projections of fright, she has become herself—a warm, enthusiastic, responsible, responsive, and consciously choosing human being.

Review quickly the progression of Rhonda's exploration of herself in her world. I see three major movements:

a little girl and a grown woman
culminating in
a seductive young woman.

From those first ventures into pieces of herself, she grew more focused and confrontive:

angry wife and angry husband
an entangled piece and an active part
panic and possibility

culminating in
    a child at the zoo and an adult at a
    museum.
From that she began to reconstruct her self-above-selves:
    an adult relationship
    some reality testing
    a temporary flight into regression
    culminating in
        limiting and loving and leaving.

Her story, like that of each of us, is not over. Her struggles will continue. There will be good days and bad days. As with each of us, she must risk becoming herself continually. . . .

3

The Case and the Key:
peace

With Rhonda's experience before us, I return to the idea of ourselves as the key to helping and being helped.

Much Eastern thought assumes that to create is to unite, to know is not to distinguish, to act is not to act: selfless self, formless form, desireless desire, noncompelling imperative, coincidence of contraries. By demolishing boundaries we allow sameness. By allowing sameness we eliminate functioning. By eliminating functioning we de-structure objects. By de-structuring objects, it is believed, we find life.

In contrast, much Western thought assumes that to create is to divide, to know is to distinguish, to act is to separate: self versus society; mind versus body; divinity versus humanity; nature versus nurture; male versus female; earth versus heaven; paradise versus purgatory; inside versus outside; conscious versus unconscious. By setting boundaries we create forms. By creating forms we generate functions. By generating functions we accumulate objects. By accumulating objects, it is believed, we find life.

But just as a sense of the one can obscure life, so we are learning that a sense of the many can likewise obliterate life. To separate one part from another part, to segregate one side from another side, to exclude some and to include others eventually leads to one-sided, lopsided, off-balance, exaggerated distortion of the oneness and wholeness that is our heritage of a divine humanity. We end up isolated and insulated in a multi-verse of our own making.

Through the centuries mystics have experienced unity within diversity, oneness in the midst of multiplicity, commonality underlying the fragmentary, affiliation at the core of alienation. Basically, outer and inner are two views of one reality. Such discovery makes for a recovery of one's genuine humanity.

The reintegrating of the pieces and parts of one's life follows an identifiable pattern.

First comes the accusation. We who have denied being out-there in the pieces are, in truth, present and active in the fragments. Out-there—in others—in objects—in events—we have involved ourselves surreptitiously. Not only have we hidden the truth from others, but also disguised it from ourselves. Now, however, being held accountable for our pervasive presence, we can say, "Yes. I am present in the pieces. I am there and there and there."

The defense follows. Having found evidence of ourselves in widely scattered pieces, we may mistakenly conclude that all of us is out-there. In point of fact, our intentions, our decisions, our efforts have been directed *against being there* in order to be here responsibly. In-here—in our consciousness—in our actions—in our attitudes—we have invested ourselves openly. We have done it conscientiously. Not only have we convinced others that this is the way we are, but we have also convinced ourselves. Now, notwithstanding, having to be explicit about our desires, we can say, "Yes. I am not only in the pieces (there and there and there), I am also in the parts (here and here and here)."

In this centering-affirmation process, temporary syntheses emerge.

We are not in the pieces out-there and we are not in the parts in-here. We are neither hidden presence nor known participant. We are more than what we have denied and other than what we have claimed.

Out-there in others—in objects—in events—we find clues to the contacting, searching, seeking, growing, uncertain, frightened, aspiring aspects of ourselves. What is missing in our here-and-now shows itself in the there-and-then. We enter into and affirm that which we have questioned as pieces of ourselves.

In-here—in our consciousness—in our actions and our attitudes—we find considerations as to the evaluating, discriminating, judging, valuing, intentional aspects of ourselves. What is missing in our there-and-then shows itself in our here-and-now. We assert and affirm that which we have stated as being parts of ourselves.

In short, neither the there-and-then of our scattered presence nor the here-and-now of our intended participation is right in and of itself. Rather, each is complementary in an ongoing process of human maturing. From the deepest perspective, each is necessary because neither is sufficient.

Now the one side; now the other.

I am present in each; I work through both
I am other than each; I am more than both
I am
I am that I am

I am there
I am there, really present, actually acting

I am here
I am here, really present, intentionally responding

I cause to be
I cause to be what comes into being

I will be what I will be . . .

living process. . . .

4

The Grammar:
common features

Sören Kierkegaard told of a philosopher who was unexpectedly confronted with his own death. The impact panicked him because his "proofs" for the immortality of the soul were in his notebook back in his study.[1]

Books on how to respond to human pain can make a difference, but in the immediate situation give-and-take gut reaction matters more. Nevertheless, even though gut reactions are crucial, it is equally important to understand the basic elements common to all helping relationships. Thus far I have emphasized starting with ourselves as the key. We are to discover the splits in our own experience. We are to recover vitality in our own many-sidedness. Now I sharpen the issue in terms of its objective structure.

What are the common features present in most, if not all, therapeutic relationships? What, in short, constitutes the grammar of responding?

The grammar of responding, like any grammar, is neat and tidy, technical and abstract. Grammar assigns order to reality. It aids us in making sense of diverse expressions.

Despite many approaches to helping, a basic grammar of responding is apparent. In fact, we are rapidly recognizing that the commonalities in interpersonal therapy "are far more impressive than their apparent differences, which may be no more than relative emphases."[2] These include such shared factors as "hope, expectation of change, trust, an emotional relationship, the facilitation of emotional arousal, catharsis, receiving information, the social impact of the healer" and so on.[3] Jerome Frank of Johns Hopkins University presents the clearest statement of the grammatical structure of interpersonal healing with which I am acquainted, and so I draw heavily upon his analysis.[4]

In seeking to understand "persuasion and healing," Frank labels the basic problem helpers face as *demoralization:* loss of spirit, a sense of failure, a feeling of powerlessness to affect oneself and one's world. A person experiences bewilderment, confusion, lack of courage. The demands of the world grow too much; the necessity to extricate oneself proves impossible. One no longer feels like dancing in one's world. Beyond demoralization as a general (nonspecific) difficulty, Frank recognizes people with specific symptoms and disturbances, but these make up only a small percentage of the sufferers who present themselves for help.

Frank goes on to wonder: regardless of whether a helper is a traditional mental health professional or a shaman in primitive society or a clergyperson or a parent or a nonmedical healer, are there features of interpersonal therapy common to all cultures? Or, as I have put the issue, what is the grammar of responding? The grammar makes explicit the formal structure and common features present in every healing approach. Understanding these features can aid us in reducing demoralization and in recovering breathing space.

A Relationship

The first feature of every therapeutic approach will not be surprising. It is bedrock: a special kind of relationship. Since the loss of significant relationships constitutes the source of demoralization, the recovery of vitality requires meaningful involvement with others. The one seeking help expects the other to be able to help. In other words, the sufferer experiences the responder as genuinely caring about his or her well-being.

When God looked out on creation, one aspect alone stood out as not good (Genesis 2:18): it is not good for humans to be alone. The pain of the therapeutic process, which, of course, is much of the pain of our human situation, compels us to ask: how can the terrible loneliness of physical proximity be transformed into the healing of personal presence?

Robert Carkhuff and Charles Truax, following the line of investigation initiated by Carl Rogers and his associates, have specified the elements of meaningful relationship more precisely. They direct us to the need for:[5]

Accurate empathy, that is, being able to know where the other person is and to let that person know that one knows. One does not invalidate the sufferer's outlook on life by reading too much into the other's world nor by discovering too little there. An interpretation that says too much may be just as disturbing for the sufferer as a reflection that says too little. Such empathic standing under another's pain provides "a strong antidote to feelings of alienation and is a potent enhancer of morale."[6] One responds sensitively and clarifyingly by words and tone and intensity to the actual in the other's presence. What lies on the surface and what lurks in the depths are genuinely disclosed. By expanding the limits of understanding, one has more options available on which to act.

Respect, which clarifies the earlier Rogerian designation of "non-possessive warmth," has two components: Unconditionality, meaning that I take you as you are where you are without qualification, deeply prizing your human potentials. Beyond this basic acceptance there lies positive regard, a regard that grows out of one's worthwhile activities and behavior. The helper actively engages the life situation of the other, taking it seriously and responding to it sensitively.

With Rhonda this relationship feature was primary. Because of previous contact, we had that going for us before our work began. She was confident that I understood both her manipulations and her strengths. Interpretations came mostly from within herself through dialogue between her several selves. As such, they felt on target. My positive regard, growing from her responsible actions, qualified my unconditional caring for her as a person. The more she chose to be who she was, the more I responded to her.

A Place

Along with a significant relationship, another common feature of every therapeutic approach is that there must be a place. To use religious language, a sanctuary is a special space that is away from one's ongoing setting. This place allows a person to come in and breathe a sigh of relief. In war that experience was labeled "R and R"—rest and recuperation. There is a space where one is away from the battle. One can let down and experience the loss of well-being. Even more, there is a place where one can take the pieces of one's life and put them together in a new and more satisfying pattern.

So, there is the psychotherapist's office or the pastor's study or the teacher's desk or "a little house of one's own." Whatever form it takes, the reality is the same—some place away from involvement where one can experience the loss of life-space and the recovering of living-room. The special boundaries of space and time are protective. By virtue of such sanctuary, one can look at rejected experience, feel "awful" feelings, try out untried behaviors, experiment with a modified or even revolutionary life-style. Regressive constraints are lifted; critical condemnation is suspended; active self-exploration predominates.

The power of the special place is rooted in the accrued experiences of humanity. Through the ages some space has mattered more than other space. Such special space was strong, significant, and, therefore, sacred. It was marked off and distinguished from other spaces. By virtue of its specialness, it was to be entered care-fully (Exodus 3:5). It is not surprising that as one approaches "the place" one experiences a quickening of attention, more rapid heartbeat, a bit of breathlessness, anxious anticipation. For the special place preeminently marks the realm of the Real. As Mircea Eliade claims, the "religious [person's] desire to live *in the sacred* is in fact equivalent to [one's] desire to take up [one's] abode in objective reality, not to let [oneself] be paralyzed by the never-ceasing relativity of purely subjective experiences, to live in a real and effective world, and not in an illusion."[7]

The belief in the temple as the *imago mundi,* that is, that "the sanctuary reproduces the universe in its essence,"[8] found architec-tural expression in the great basilicas and medieval cathedrals.

The special place always symbolized the Center. It marked the meeting point of heaven, earth, and hell. Mythically, the summit of the cosmic mountain marked both the highest point of earth and also earth's navel, the point at which creation originated.

Thus, the sanctuary allows passage from one realm to another, from the vibrant underground to the controlled ordinariness to the ecstatic transcendent. Here is the realm of the Real. But the passage, the road, the way leading to the sacred place is always fraught with difficulty. Because of the transition from the profane to the sacred, from the illusion to reality, from time to eternity, from death to life, from chaos to cosmos, the way is perilous.

To be in the special place—the space of the Center—one comes to experience a fixed and focused orientation. In the midst of the disruptive, one discovers order. The entrance into the special place constitutes the boundary line between inner and outer reality. It sets the limit that distinguishes the chaos of the passing from the orderliness of the permanent.

Yet the entrance also, paradoxically, expresses the coincidence of opposites. It is the place where the world of pain and the world of healing meet. The foreign, strange, unknown, meaningless, threatening realm of the transient begins to be inhabited and possessed. To dwell in one's previously rejected experience is equivalent to founding a new world, to entering into a new life.[9]

"In the last analysis," Eliade concludes, *"it is by virtue of the temple that the world is resanctified in every part."*[10] The special place reduces and eventually destroys the arbitrary distinction between the safety of the sanctuary and the threat of the world. The world once again reveals itself as cosmos, as ordered, as oriented, as sacred, as really real.

With Rhonda this special space assumed crucial significance. The office at the Counseling Center served to protect us from uncontrollable emotion. There she had to face what she feared, yet felt shielded from its consequence. The center gave her a place to experience the pieces, to explore the parts, and to integrate her several selves.

A Rationale

Remember that I am spelling out the grammar of therapeutic approaches. As such, the process is logical. Remember also that these features intertwine. They are separable only for analysis.

A rationale provides a way of naming the reality with which one is contending. In Jesus' encounter with the man possessed by demons, he asked, "What is your name?" The answer was, "My name is Legion, for I am in many pieces" (see Mark 5:1-20). As soon as the man was able to label and thereby identify his experience, he began to recover his peace.

For healing to occur, it is never enough simply to experience caring. Neither is it enough to have a place. We need some way of recognizing or assigning meaning to what is happening. Thus, in growth groups there is the constant emphasis:

"Can you *say* what you're feeling?"

"Can you *name* your experience?"

"Let me try to put into words what I sense you're feeling. . . . Is this right?"

And so the struggle to bring together just the right expression for the very real experience goes on.

Morton Liebermann, Irvin Yalom, and Matthew Miles conducted a comprehensive investigation of sixteen encounter groups and their leaders. They compared the approaches and assessed the outcomes. For my purposes I want to deal only with what they found as to leader behavior and its impact.

Differences in how the leaders worked could not be related to differences in their theoretical orientations. Instead, four basic leadership functions emerged. These underlie various leader behaviors. They are:

1. *Emotional Stimulation:* emphasizing disclosing feelings, attitudes, beliefs, and values; challenging, confronting, participating;
2. *Caring:* expressing warmth, acceptance, genuineness, concern;
3. *Meaning-Attribution:* providing concepts and frameworks for understanding, clarifying, interpreting, naming, and giving meaning to experience;
4. *Executive Function:* limit setting and directing.[11]

Analysis of the impact of the leader on participant outcome in terms of these functions was clear. The most effective style was associated with high caring and the utilization of meaning-attribution plus moderate stimulation and executive function. Either too much or too little stimulation and executive function were associated with negative outcomes.

Meaning-attribution or language does not simply order experience. It is also part and parcel of a whole structure of the way the world is met and mastered, contacted and created. Rationales of healing explain the cause of a sufferer's pain; they spell out desirable goals for the person; they outline procedures for attaining these goals. Built into the rationales—or myths as Frank terms them—is an implicit optimism about life. One need not be as pained as one is; one can be relieved of one's symptoms; even more, one can be restored to the land of living and loving relationships. Demoralization can be defeated!

Transactional analysis (TA) is one rationale currently used. It began with Eric Berne and *Games People Play*. It attained notoriety with Thomas Harris and *I'm OK—You're OK*. It provides a convenient map of human interaction. Simple, yes; yet, nevertheless, sensible.

In the system it is postulated that everyone has three ego states: the Parent, the Adult, and the Child.

The adult ego state deals with reality in a straightforward way. The parental ego state is divided into contrasting pairs: the good parent, the nurturing parent, the generative parent (in Erikson's developmental scheme) *and* the critical parent, the condemning parent, the one whose expectations (or what we take to be the expectations) we somehow can never live up to. The child ego state also divides into contrasting pairs: the positive quality of being childlike, the delightful, the Nasrudin-like, the one who is free enough to be foolish *and* the brat, the person who pouts, Ahab going into his room and turning his face to the wall and sulking, the parasite who just wants to take and take and take from the environment without giving anything in turn.

With that rationale in mind, we can apply it to the way we communicate. I hope that at this point in the book we have the adult-to-adult contact. More precisely, I may be a capital *A*dult and you may be a lower case *a*dult, but if we were talking together, there would be moments when you would be instructing me and I would be learning from you. Then the capital *A*dult and the lower case *a*dult would be reversed, according to the circumstances.

One expression of the various ego states is the way we scramble normal communication. For instance, I return home at night, say from a hard day, and drag into the kitchen, slouch down at the table, and do not say anything. I simply sit there—really—as a child. I am not behaving as an adult-child. That is, I do not take responsibility for what I am experiencing. Instead, I want my wife to attend to my needs *without* my having to tell her that I want her to take care of me. The message goes from child to parent: "Be a good mother to me. Ask me, 'Jim, how did it go today? You look pretty weary.'"

But she is standing at the sink working on supper. She has had a hard day, scrambling with fifty kids and a staff of ten as director of a day care center. She sends out a similar message only in reverse. She wants me to ask her, "Honey, how did it go today? It must have been really rough. You look done in." She wants me to be a nurturing parent.

Such scrambled messages seldom meet except in terms of noisy confusion. She feels: "What have I done now? Why is he angry with me?" I feel: "I'm let down again. She doesn't love me." Such contact does not exactly make for dancing.

Transactional analysis provides a grammar with which people can dissect such scrambled messages in order to make sense of the pain. The analysis enables us to identify that "I am being a sulking kid" and "you are feeling like a naughty child." We both then "see" that what we want is not the conflict but the caring. When I come to realize that I must take responsibility for wanting to be a child, then I can say, "Honey, I need a little loving right now." In turn, when she comes to realize that she wants to be a child, then she can say, "I want a little loving myself." Those are clear messages.

With that she can say to me, "I'm too busy to give it to you now. Wait until 8:30." Or, if I were really liberated and in the kitchen getting supper, I could say, "I'm too busy now. How about 8:30?"

Thus, TA is a way of looking at behavior, just as is Timothy Leary's interpersonal diagnosis of personality (which I describe systematically in the chapter on dependency) or Gestalt theory which I used with Rhonda or Jungian theory or Freudian theory or behavior modification theory. It does not matter so much *what* the rationale or meaning-attribution may be, as long as it provides some kind of structure that connects inner experience and outer behavior in a systematic and sensible way.

Lieberman, Yalom, and Miles found in their study that cognitive factors play a "far more important [role] in producing positive outcome in encounter groups than is generally realized." No conceptual scheme appeared more or less effective than any other. Instead, what members learned was "a general strategy which they could employ in understanding and resolving problematic areas. They were able to assume a diagnostic observing stance toward important life dilemmas. The specific types of coping strategies internalized were at times disarmingly simple. What seemed to be the most important thing was that people whom they had grown to respect (the leaders and other members of the group) advocated a reflective, self-conscious attitude toward coping." [12]

I regard psychological rationale in the same way as theological rationale. Theology is a systematic way of expressing and organizing the experience of the worshiping community. But, for me, there can be no official theology. No theory adequately expresses the experience which it seeks to reflect; every theory creates and discloses much of that experience. Some rationale or meaning-attribution *is* necessary. But to insist upon one and only one rationale turns varied expressions into propaganda.

Evocative or insight-oriented therapies emphasize general demoralization while minimizing specific symptoms. By deepening the sufferer's inner freedom via self-knowledge, the person becomes more spontaneous, with resulting satisfaction and success. Once the person is inwardly less constricted, development will continue by itself. The main object of treatment, however, is "not so much surcease of pain as the establishment of a context of meaning in life of which the pain is an intelligible part." [13]

Directive or action-oriented therapies shift the emphasis from general demoralization to specific pain. By aiding the sufferer to regain his or her sense of control, the helper alleviates the present complaints. Once the person is freed from the symptoms, development will continue by itself. No purpose is gained by explaining behavior, according to these approaches. What matters is learning how to control and modify specific behaviors. [14]

With Rhonda I combined elements of communication and Gestalt theories. The rationale reduced the chaos of her experiences by offering ways to identify what was happening. Her unknown inner world gradually turned into a known habitation. We dealt with her general disorganization through exploration of her specific concerns. The rationale activated her ability to think helpfully about herself.

In the immediacy of responding there is what Perry London observed as "a quiet blending of techniques by artful therapists of [whatever] school; a blending that takes account of the fact that people are considerably simpler than the Insight schools give them credit for, but that they are also more complicated than the Action therapists would like to believe." [15]

Procedures

Within every therapeutic style there develops a procedure or a strategy consistent with the rationale which is designed to help the sufferer. By means of it one receives new information about oneself.

One tries out new experiencing of and different interacting with the world. Here, then, is the fourth common feature.

One therapist friend has a tactic when he feels himself entangled in self-defeating interaction with clients. He gets up and has his client get up and they walk around the room. This way he seeks to unscramble the associative chain in hopes of allowing other interaction to emerge. By breaking up a negative gestalt, more constructive ones are disclosed.

Every relationship has a procedural grammar to feed in new ideas and new experience. In the safety of the special place one can try out expressions that might not be tried outside. In the protection of "this place" it is all right to experience the fact that one really did—in a moment of intense reality—hate one's mother for having given one a chaotic world. In the protection of "this place" it is all right to recover that resentment—to reown and repossess it—to finish it by remembering now in order to forget what previously one had forgotten to remember. On the other side of the negative, one can find the blessing: instead of conventionality, her gift has been creativity!

We need procedures that allow us to put different labels on old experiences. Again and again those who tag certain experiences "bad" are liberated when they discover that within those very experiences lie the positive and the creative and the "good."

The procedures, no matter how varied, require active participation by the helper as well as the sufferer. Whenever healing comes, there is always genuine involvement by the caring person. That does not mean necessarily a warm, friendly helper. Many confuse active participation with warmth and friendliness, but more of that later. Rather, active helper involvement means serious engagement in the interaction, caring passionately yet nonpossessively about the other and where the other is.

For the sufferer, the procedures serve various functions. They encourage one to try out different ways of coming at the world. By virtue of their orderliness, the methods quicken one's hope of relief. At the same time the methods enhance one's coping skill and interpersonal competence. A more positive self-image replaces a negative self-image. One is aroused to engage the painful with confidence—relief and healing will come.

With Rhonda the technique of being one's projection (as the primary one I am emphasizing here) had several consequences. She could enter into deeper and different experiencing. She could try out more and varied communications. She discovered ranges of feelings of which she had been only dimly aware. She realized priorities of values which had only been in conflict and chaos. She acted in ways that let her learn from her behavior, sorting out the more desirable from the less desirable. She found *she* could be in charge of her life so as to become more herself.

These elements, then, make up the grammar of the helping situation: a special relationship, a special place, a rationale, systematic procedures. Caring *and* cognitive structure are both needed. But they do not guarantee healing. The grammatical structure must contain meaningful experience. Not the bare bones, but genuine relatedness—interpersonally and intrapsychically—is vital.

5

The Whole Person: body and brain

Thus far I have stressed interpersonal and intrapsychic dimensions of responding to human pain. While I do not reduce these dimensions to our bodies, I do find recent research suggesting bodily processes and structures to which these are relatable, if not related. At the very least, such processes and structures help me link the various dimensions with each other.

Specifically, I find Hans Selye's work on the biological basis of stress and Robert Ornstein's interpretation of the brain fruitful in understanding the ways we function. In understanding bodily stress and the workings of the brain, I find I can respond more helpfully to human pain.

Bodily Stress

Stress can no longer be regarded as a typical response to events or pressure from outside nor as the specific result of particular actions of our own. Instead, it is "a common feature of all biological activities." The magnitude of stress can be determined by measurable effects upon the body, specifically in such functions as: adrenal stimulation, shrinkage of lymphatic organs, gastrointestinal ulcers, loss of body weight, and alterations in the chemical composition of the body.[1]

This configuration of bodily features is called the general adaption syndrome because of its three states. It is:

—*general* because only agents having a general effect upon large portions of the body produce it;

—*adaptive* because it stimulates defense and thereby helps the body acquire and maintain a stage of accommodation;

—a *syndrome* "because its individual manifestations are coordinated and even partly dependent upon each other."[2]

All three elements are necessary for a state of stress to exist. What Selye has demonstrated is that "stress is an essential element of all our actions, in health and in disease."[3] When stress is absent, life is absent. When stress is present, life is present.

Hippocrates suggested that disease is not only suffering or *pathos* but also toil or *pónos*. That is, the body fights to restore itself toward the normal. "Disease is not mere surrender to disease, but also fight for health; and unless there is fight there is no disease." Contrast this to the person born with a physical handicap. In such a condition "there is no *pónos,* no toil; the fight was lost long ago and now there is peace in the body, although it is a scarred body."[4]

Stress equalizes bodily activities. It prevents overexertion in either work or rest.[5] If you are carrying a heavy suitcase with one arm, fatigue sets in rapidly. Fatigue is a sign of local stress and calls for change. "If there is proportionately too much stress in any one part," Selye counsels, "you need diversion. If there is too much stress in the body as a whole, you must rest."[6] "Nature likes variety. . . . if you use the same parts of your body or mind over and over again, the only means nature has to force you out of the groove is: stress."[7]

The essence of stress may be understood as a three-stage process:

1. the *alarm* that something is wrong,
2. the *resistance* of the organism to that malfunctioning, and
3. the *submission* of the organism to the condition.[8]

I am struck by the parallel with the process of pieces and parts transformed into peace. The initial shock of recognition comes in the alarm that something is wrong. The middle confrontation of intentions shows our resistance to what is upsetting. The final recognition of choices appears with submission to the situation.

Evocative or insight-oriented therapies focus on general stress while minimizing specific symptoms. They are dealing with the general alarm system that alerts the whole body to the assault of stress. As the person grows more aware of influences and choices, the alarm system no longer goes off at the slightest stress. One is more oneself and so can deal with stressful situations with appropriately circumscribed discriminations.

Directive or action-oriented therapies shift the focus from the general to the specific. By aiding the sufferer to regain control, the helper alleviates the presenting complaints. Stress is resisted with the least expenditure of the person's energy. Once the person is freed from the specific symptoms triggering the general alarm, general stress disappears. One is more able to do what one wants because appropriate energy is available.

The concept of stress as Selye develops it provides a biological analogue for the dialectic dynamic of pieces and parts. The movement proceeds from alarm and the shock of recognition to resistance and the confrontation of intentions to submission and the recognition of choices. This last phase is resolution of the unexpected stress of the first phase and the intentional stress of the middle phase.

The Brain

The brain presents us with an even clearer bodily analogue to the dynamics of being and becoming oneself. The contrast between experiencing ourselves *as* everything and expressing ourselves *in* everything appears to have a physiological basis. This differentiation of "as" and "is" arises, I am convinced, because each of us possesses one brain with two parts. Indirectly, we have "known" that for centuries, as seen in people's experiences of contrasts and opposites, dichotomies and dualities. Now we are accumulating evidence to support the physiological base of the polarities in human understanding.

Roger Bacon, for instance, in 1268, described two ways of knowing: knowledge by argument and knowledge by experience. Knowledge by argument consisted of articulate, reasonable, analytical, sequential, and active thinking. Knowledge by experience included sensuous, spatial, holistic, relational, and receptive experience.[9]

When people are asked to reflect on different sides of their bodies—right and left—a similar contrast emerges.[10] Most experience the right side as stronger and the left side as weaker. Around the strength people report a constellation of such qualities as masculine, active, logical, mechanical, and "light." Around the weakness they report such qualities as feminine, passive, intuitive, artistic, and "dark." The two sides are not equal in their meaning; they are separate and distinct. The right side tends to be more familiar and decisive. The left side tends to be less familiar and indecisive. The two parts of the brain reflect these contrasts in consciousness and activity.[11] Let me elaborate more specifically.

The left hemisphere functions on the right side of the body. It includes the active, shaping, initiating, intentional aspects of consciousness and activity. Physiologically, it involves the large striate muscles and the sympathetic nervous system. Psychologically, it shows itself in focal attention, achievement, sharp boundaries, clear distinctions, striving, and shaping. Its goal is acting on the world and making it in the world. It is oriented to time and the future. Language, verbal capacity, mathematics, science, and formal logic comprise its activity. If you think of a taxi driver rushing through traffic to get you to the airport when you are late for a plane, you have some sense of the way the left hemisphere works. It is the "right" hand grasp, the correct response, the ability to attain a clearly determined goal. One is more protected, less accessible, less open to similarities and commonalities, more opposed and distant.

The right hemisphere, in contrast, functions on the left side of the body. It includes the receptive, being shaped by and being responsive to the environment, taking in what is round about, the marginal and peripheral aspects of consciousness and activity. Physiologically, it involves sensory awareness and the autonomic nervous system. Psychologically, it shows itself in peripheral and diffused attention, decrease in boundary perception, increase in the sensory and paralogical thought processes (over the formal ones), the artistic, the musical, the motoric, the ability to recognize faces. Its goal is letting happen and taking in what is. It is oriented to space, the simultaneous, and the relational. If you think of someone meditating quietly, letting go of all focused thought, freeing oneself from pursuing any particular thought, emptying one's awareness of specific content, you have some sense of the way the right hemisphere works. It is the "left" hand touch, the awkward, subtle, gentler response, the sensitive ability to resonate with what is. One is more vulnerable, more accessible, more open to blurring boundaries and distinctions, more connected and closer.

The left hemisphere may be regarded as the active, intellectual expression of "I want." The right hemisphere may be regarded as the receptive, intuitive experience of "I am." In the assertive response, life tends to be simpler and more concrete. In picturing the difference between the two sides of the brain, the *Sunday New York Times Magazine Section* showed a human head. On the left side was a page from a dictionary with the various definitions of the word "dance." On the right was the Degas picture of two ballerinas dancing.[12]

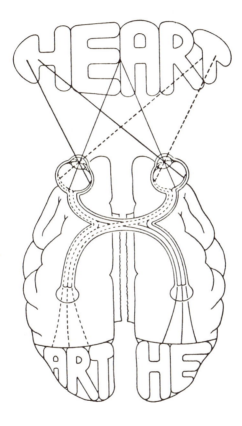

FIGURE 5.1
A simplified diagram of visual input to the two hemispheres of the brain. Images in the left visual field are projected to the right hemisphere, images in the right visual field to the left hemisphere. This schematic drawing illustrates one experiment performed on split-brain patients: note that the corpus callosum is cut. The "HE" and "ART" projections are, of course, fanciful, not anatomically correct.

From *The Psychology of Consciousness* by Robert E. Ornstein. W. H. Freeman and Company. Copyright © 1972.

Each hemisphere operates independently of the other. Each is unique, separate, distinguishable. Yet they are held together and coordinated by connecting fibers known as the corpus callosum. The corpus callosum may be thought of as the lines of communication between one side of the brain and the other, conveying messages back and forth. There is feedback between the two sides, thereby integrating information into an intentional whole.

In recent years a number of people have been found who, whether as the result of an accident or of special surgery, have had those connecting fibers severed. Thus, they are labeled "split-brain" people.[13] These people have two independent brains, each functioning separately from the other. Experiments with "split-brain" people and normal people have begun to produce data about the way our brains work and implications for the way we act.

In one experiment, split-brain patients saw the letters HEART flashed on a screen. They were asked to say what they saw, in other words, to respond from the left hemisphere. All of them reported: "I saw the word ART." Then they were instructed to point with their left hand to what they saw; in other words, to respond from the right hemisphere. All of them pointed to HE. Figure 5.1 shows the visual input to the two hemispheres where the corpus callosum is cut.

Different answers are given to the same question. Verbally, they gave one response to what they saw. Nonverbally, they gave another. In other experiments, split-brain people could spell words with their left hands when they were unable to say what they spelled.

The right hemisphere is limited in its overall command of language. Although it can respond to a concrete noun such as "pencil," it has more difficulty with verbs, for example, not responding to simple printed instructions such as "smile" or "frown." Its poorly developed grammatical sense is suggested by its inability to form the plural of a given word. At the same time the right hemisphere excels in such tasks as arranging blocks to match a pictured design or drawing a cube in three dimensions as seen in Figure 5.2. In another experiment, split-brain patients were given a square to copy. When drawing with the right hand, they might draw the four corners stacked together. They only drew the corners but not the connections. When drawing with the left hand, they copied spatial figures but not a written word.

The two hemispheres function separately but not simultaneously. When one side is active, the other is quiet. That has been ascertained by brain wave reaction patterns. In activation there is a decrease in

EXAMPLE   LEFT HAND   RIGHT HAND

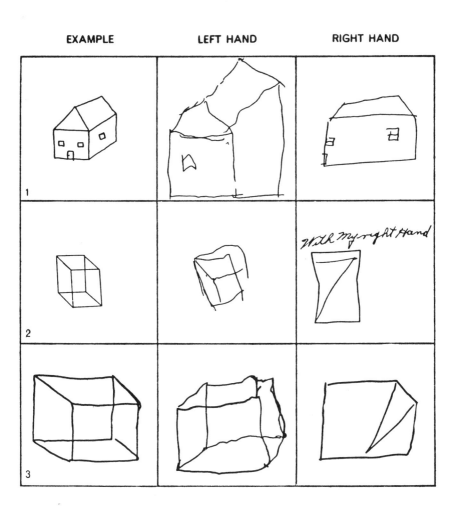

FIGURE 5.2
"Visual-constructional" tasks are handled better by the right hemisphere. **This was seen most clearly in the first patient, who had poor ipsilateral control of his right hand.** Although righthanded, he could copy the examples only with his left hand.

the alpha waves; in rest there is an increase in the alpha waves.

The left hemisphere and the right side are linked with control of the voluntary nervous system. The assertive, aggressive initiative comes out in active volition for the sake of biological and individual survival. Think of this metaphorically as the presence of the bright light of the sun.

The right hemisphere and the left side are linked with control of the autonomic nervous system. The receptive, unresistive taking-in comes out in passive volition for the sake of sociological and spiritual survival. Think of this metaphorically as the presence of the subtle light of the stars.

In active volition we tense the body, brace ourselves, tighten up to meet a challenge. In passive volition we relax the body, detach ourselves, let go of effort to be part of what is.

Frederick Franck points to the contrast when he draws and writes of "seeing/drawing as meditation":

> Looking and seeing both start with sense perception, but there the similarity ends. When I "look" at the world and label its phenomena, I make immediate choices, instant appraisals—I like or I dislike, I accept or reject, what I look at, according to its usefulness to the "Me" . . . THIS ME THAT I IMAGINE MYSELF TO BE, and that I try to impose on others.
> The purpose of "looking" is to survive, to cope, to manipulate, to discern what is useful, agreeable, or threatening to the Me, what enhances or what diminishes the Me. This we are trained to do from our first day.
> When, on the other hand, I SEE—suddenly I am all eyes, I forget this Me, am liberated from it and dive into the reality of what confronts me, become part of it, participate in it. I no longer label, no longer choose. . . .[14]

Lancelot Whyte contends that European thinkers have tended to fall into two camps: "the one seeking order, similarities, and unity (often called 'mystical' or 'religious') and the other differences between particulars (the 'tough' thinkers or scientists). The first seek comfort in feeling a unifying order, the second in defining of particulars."[15] Antagonism between the two has been so intense at times that members from one camp have scarcely spoken to those of the other camp. Yet each side represents what the other has inhibited yet used unconsciously.

Evocative or insight-oriented therapies draw upon the holistic and integrating capacity of the right hemisphere. They seek contact with the experiential ground of personhood. By seeing—the "ahah" of the gestalt discovery in which chaos turns into cosmos—a person reconstrues his or her world creatively. One is in tune with what is.

Directive or action-oriented therapies rely upon the analytical and discriminating capacity of the left hemisphere. They seek clarification of specific stress and the application of specific behaviors. By looking, a person acts in his or her world constructively. One sets the tone for what can be.

Life requires both parts of our brain. Each is necessary; neither is sufficient. The strength of one compensates for and complements the limitation of the other. While in extreme circumstances it is possible to function with only one hemisphere, most of the time each counterbalances the one-sidedness of the other. We create by actively putting out into the world that which is successive, discrete, individual. We center by receptively taking in from the world that which is simultaneous, diffuse, collective.

In responding to human need, investigation has identified common features in the various therapeutic approaches. We found in examining the grammar that the features could be reduced to two.

One is caring or the connecting relationship, which I relate to the right hemisphere and its functioning. Here is identification with that which is, the supporting setting, the humanness of another, the everlasting arms. I call this the logic of the marginal and the peripheral. It is the variable of being.

The other is cognitive structure or some logical way of organizing the environment to make sense of one's experience, which I relate to the left hemisphere and its functioning. Love is not enough; caring is not sufficient. Naming, language, creating, identifying, making distinctions (as in Genesis 2 and 3) are also necessary. Without these a person lacks skills and competence in engaging the world efficiently and effectively. I call this the logic of the focused and the central. It is the variable of doing.

Coming at human nature from a similar direction, David Bakan explores what he calls *The Duality of Human Existence*. For him the essential duality is between the modality of agency for the existence of the individual and the modality of communion for the participation of the individual in a larger whole. Agency includes: (1) self-protection, self-assertion, and self-expansion; (2) the formation of separations; (3) isolation, alienation, and aloneness; (4) the urge to master; and (5) repression of thought, feeling, and impulse.[16] Obviously, this constellation goes with left hemisphere activity. Communion includes these contrasts: (1) the sense of being at one with other organisms; (2) the lack of separations; (3) contact, openness, and union; (4) noncontractual cooperation; (5) the lack and removal of repression. Again, this constellation relates to hemisphere activity, in this case the right hemisphere.

All of this is to suggest that both parts of the brain and both sides of ourselves are necessary if we are to be whole persons.

Neither the active side nor the receptive side is sufficient to create the whole. To get oneself together, each side is necessary. We are made for active engagement *and* receptive involvement.

None of us ends in ourself; none of us begins with ourself. The fulfillment of meaning is always more than the fulfillment of me. As Paul claimed, "For though everything belongs to you . . . the world, life, and death, the present and the future, all of them belong to you— yet you belong to Christ, and Christ to God" (1 Corinthians 3:21-23, NEB). The structure of our being both reflects *and* creates our world. Yet the structure is not of "our" making; it is the Logos, the orderly structuring of the uni-verse, of everything that is.

In one place Meister Eckhart was talking about the chaos of the margin, the underground, or however one wants to name it. He then declared, ". . . In bursting forth I discover that God and I are One. Now I am what I was [meant to be]."[17]

Most people who write and read books like this carry responsibility in society. We tend, consequently, to be those who emphasize too much order, too much control, too much regularity, too much active willing. Now, because of our technology, we are catching up with the visionaries from the past. We are learning that we *can* burst forth, not in terms of the destructive, but in terms of discovery. We are recovering the wholeness of our world—of others, of ourselves, of humanity.

As we get ourselves together, we can give ourselves to where we are. We criticize what-is-not and we celebrate what-is. We criticize what-is and we celebrate what-is-not. We uproot and we reroot. We work and we love. The key lies within ourselves as whole persons.

6

The Guts:
personal demands

I have been setting down the structure and procedures for responding. In this has been the assumption of unquestioned responsiveness. Before turning to more specific expressions of pain in the next section, we need to step back and take a hard look at the personal demands confronting the person who would respond. Instead of looking outward, we are to look inward. While we ourselves are still the key, the inward look now serves a different purpose, namely, asking "Am I able to respond?"

"There are many people," Kierkegaard observed, "who reach their conclusions about life like school[children]: they cheat their master by copying the answer out of a book without having worked the sum out for themselves."[1] Personal demands can be sensed in three basic questions.[2] These questions focus the issue of our having to face aspects of ourselves whenever we respond to others' pain. In the other I am forced to see myself.

As I indicated above, it is important to distinguish between what is clearly the other's and what I find of myself in the other. In empathy I see in the other what is of the other. In sympathy I find in the other what is of my own. If I show only empathy, I have created the illusory divorce of "me" and "not me." Similarly, if I show only sympathy, I have created the delusory narcissism that the world is only an extension of "me." Sympathetic empathy allows me to see the other "as other" without alienation. Empathetic sympathy encourages me to see the other "as of common essence" without absorption. Both personal sympathy—the caring of the right hemisphere—and objective empathy—the cognitive structuring of the left hemisphere—are needed.

Do I Want to Help?

The first demand is movement toward others. Do I *really* want to help?

That sounds like a simple question. Of course I want to help—in the abstract, above the messy give-and-take of immediate need. But I find that when I am with hostile, demanding, domineering, smothering, dependent, clinging, passive-aggressive people, I wonder whether I really do want to help. The feeling is analogous to that expressed by our youngest daughter when she announced, "I enjoy hiking; it is just that I don't like to walk."

That is, do I genuinely intend movement toward and contact with people in pain? Am I prepared for real engagement?

No one ought to answer that question quickly. Do I really want to put myself at the disposal of other people's needs and to put my own real needs aside? Do I want to show genuine respect for others no matter how obnoxious they may be and no matter how much garbage may come my way? I have to ask whether or not I am prepared to experience and face failure. Others may not want me to be at their disposal. They may not accept my good intentions and genuine respect. They may use me in ways that are self-defeating for them and exploitative of me. They may never do their own work.

One needs to ask this question of wanting to help *before* one enters into responding relationships. Otherwise feelings of disappointment and resentment creep in. "They don't appreciate all I am doing for them. If they did, they would change as I want them to change. Also, they would like me." Such feelings in a helping person reflect "the inner child of the past" behind the mask of a nurturing parent.

Am I genuinely wanting and willing to risk the peace of my life for the pieces of others' lives? Am I really prepared to experience the disturbing depths of others' turmoil? I have to ask whether I am prepared—really—to manifest intelligent, outgoing concern for others' well-being independent of my own. Irrespective of others' responses, irrespective of others' appreciation, irrespective of others' resentment, I have to ask whether I am ready to face others. For I can only face in others what I am able to face in myself.

There are no textbook answers to such probings. There are only our individually determined decisions.

For myself, there are circumstances when I do not want to help. There are some people with whom I do not care to work. I find marital therapy, for instance, generally too demanding. I prefer not to see both partners at the same time in the same place, even though I "know" that is the better strategy. My own personal history intensifies that kind of conflict for me unnecessarily. I am not prepared *in myself* to deal with the depths of the stress between partners in that way.

There are periods when I do not care to respond. Sometimes I find myself so exhausted I am unable to mobilize more than a grouchy resentment and a rumbling irritation. Those are times when I become selectively inattentive to others' pain. My own needs take priority. I must take time to get myself together. I have gotten out of touch with myself by giving myself away too much. I respond only so long and then I have to *not* respond.

So be prepared, whenever others come, to ask yourself whether you really want to help. Have some sense of whether you are ready to risk opening yourself to the depths of others' disturbance.

Am I Tough Enough to Help?

Though similar, a second question focuses on a more active aspect of responding: Am I tough enough to help? That is, can the path of my life go against the paths of others' lives? Instead of an endless "Yes . . ." there comes some kind of confrontation, some kind of over-againstness, some kind of limit setting, some kind of "No!"

Am I prepared—really—to face others' realities, to risk others' anger, to allow others' separateness? In other words, am I able to stand firm in the presence of others' failures or frenzy or fearfulness and to sharpen what is the truth of the situation? Am I able to put aside winning and losing in a relationship and understand the frustrations as well as the possibilities?

In the ordinary ways we think of love, love is not enough. "The attempt to keep the relationship on a pleasant level is one of the greatest sources of ineffectual helping," declares Alan Keith-Lucas.[3] If I foster only likeness and closeness, I obscure differences and distances. With likeness and closeness we establish identification; with differences and distances we encourage identity and individuality. By reminding sufferers and ourselves of differences and distance, we prevent a misuse of the relationship by both the helper and the one seeking help. With empathic caring I provide an occasion for others to see discrepancies and contradictions and self-defeating patterns. Reality provides the context of growth.

To be tough is to confront. Confrontation brings to the fore discordant differences between the helper and the sufferer. It precipitates a self-exploration which eventually leads to a more intentional direction. Confrontation occurs whenever a sufferer expresses himself or herself one way and the helper experiences and describes the same situation in a different way. Rather than interpreting or explaining, the helper focuses on his or her own experiencing of the situation. Two excerpts suggest how a discrepancy is made explicit.

> *Client:* I'm a cool guy. I really think I'm great.... You can tell by the way I dress and talk . . . I'm just cool.
> *Therapist:* You speak of yourself as being a pretty good guy, but I guess you don't believe it or you wouldn't say it so loud and so often.

> *Client:* Now that I see what my father has done to me all these years, I feel like a new man.
> *Therapist:* Yes, but you're still getting up at 6 AM to cater to his requests just like you always did.[4]

In analyzing the effects of confrontation, Susan Anderson found that therapists rated as high in the facilitative conditions of empathy, positive regard, genuineness, concreteness, and self-disclosure had "a significantly greater tendency to confront than did therapists rated low" in these conditions. In addition, low-rated therapists "confronted clients more often with their limitations than with their resources, while high therapists tended to confront clients more often with resources."[5] That is, high-rated therapists directed attention to the ignored and denied and rejected strengths of the sufferer.

One qualification of this pattern must be noted. College students tended to explore themselves more deeply when faced with discrepancies directed to their limitations rather than their strengths. It may be that students have been burdened by an overemphasis on their potential and feel a lack of substance in their strengths.

When confrontation emerges in a caring relationship, the sufferer receives it as an expression of respect for his or her strength as a person. If you have your arms around others, you can hit them as hard as you want without hurting them. If you do not have your arms around others, the slightest brush of a feather will knock them over.

Can I stand against others' unsatisfying but "safe" behavior? Can I generate constructive anxiety by not allowing others to continue self-defeating ways?

Here is a young woman, about twenty-two, who comes for relief of interpersonal pain. In the process of her telling me about her distress, I experience myself being flooded with words. I feel I am drowning under a torrential flood of verbiage. As a polite person, I wait for a pause to get a word in edgewise, yet no pause comes. Twenty years ago when that occurred, it took me twenty minutes to move against the flood, to interrupt the pain. Today I would move in quickly, simply because with experience and a rationale I am able to make inferences from a little data more rapidly.

Finally I said to her, "Stop."

She kept on. . . .

"STop."

She kept on. . . .

"STOp."

She kept on. . . .

"STOP! STOP! STOP!" One has to be a bit dramatic in such situations. There has to be something forceful enough to arrest the pressure.

Well, she stopped, finally, and started again.

"No, no. Stop! Stop!" Then I continued, "Now start every sentence by saying, 'Jim, I . . .' and finish the sentence with whatever comes to your mind."

A simple suggestion. Nothing extraordinary. Certainly not profound. Only, "Jim, I. . . ."

For ten minutes I was harangued on what first names meant. Being slower in those days, I took longer to get untangled. Eventually, I went on, "Come on, now. Here I am and here you are. We are both here in this safe place [and I am giving you accurate empathy and unconditional positive regard and all that stuff]. Just talk with me as an old friend and say, 'Jim, I . . .' and go on to say something to me."

"Jim, I. . . ." Her words came across as mechanical, lifeless, empty.

"No, no. That's no good."

"Jim, I. . . ." More of the same.

"No! Speak to *me*."

I cannot reproduce on paper the sounds that came, but she began speaking *to* me. "Jim, I. . . ." Suddenly she started weeping. For many minutes she sobbed and sobbed and sobbed. Then came the painful, yet genuine, words, "Jim, I don't know what to say. I don't know what to say."

Interrupting the defensive pattern, being tough enough to stop maladaptive behavior, is seldom easy. That uncreative suffering is what Paul (2 Corinthians 7:10) would call "worldly" sorrow in contrast to "Godly" sorrow. Worldly sorrow, as I see it, means endless turmoil without healing. Godly sorrow means suffering that makes for healing. To stop aggression one must be aggressive in an aggressively nonaggressive way. To explode apathy one must be indifferent in an apathetically nonapathetic way. The only way out of extreme withdrawnness is via angry outburst. Am I tough enough to have my path go against the paths of others?

Do I have enough identity and integrity of my own, as Carl Rogers puts it, not to be downcast by others' depression nor sucked in by others' dependency nor frightened by others' anxieties?[6] In other words, are my ego boundaries clear enough that I can stand against others' ego boundaries (or lack thereof)?

One must not answer that question of toughness too easily.

Am I Humble Enough to Help?

A final question that personally confronts the helper is: Am I humble enough to help? Do I have enough life of my own so that I do not need to exploit the lives of others? That is, am I big enough not to have to be all?

Reinhold Niebuhr once observed that many people play God so much of the time they end up being the devil.[7] We must continually pray, "Forgive us our possessing as we forgive those who have tried to possess us." Am I humble enough to know that my life is never big enough to bear the full weight of others' lives?

Can I allow others to fail without having it undermine my own life? Can I allow others to find their own satisfaction without having to draw upon that for my own satisfaction?

If my need to help others is a disguised expression of my own uncertainties, then I exploit others by making them into extensions of myself. I use them to support me and my needs. Thus, I have to ask whether I can genuinely free others from my own emotions and prejudices. Can I allow others the freedom to be who they are and to become what they intend?

My way can never be *the* way. My reality is always so much less than the larger reality of which I am only a part.

A major trap in our desire to help is that of helping too much. "One of the conditions under which help can be given," insists Alan Keith-Lucas, "must be that the helper does not too passionately wish to give it. This does not mean that [one] is indifferent or does not care. It means that [one] cares so much that the help given is real help that [one] will not insist on it being given when it is inappropriate."[8]

I must give up moving into another's life-space. In biblical imagery, Moses sees the Promised Land yet does not enter it (Deuteronomy 32:52). Jesus says "I must go away if you are to receive the Comforter" (see John 16:7-8). Present reality is crucified for the sake of an unknown future reality. Reproduction in spirit depends upon an interruption in continuity.[9]

I am to give up my need to be needed. I am to let go of my desire for others to be like me. I am to decrease that others may increase. My movement is to be apart from the movement of others. I am to be a servant even as I do not allow myself to be mastered.[10]

Growth never comes at the same rate or in the same way for every person. So our paths intersect and our paths move against each other and our paths move apart. We can be grateful when physical closeness changes into personal presence. We know what it is to be together. We then can become those selves which we truly are.

The deepest demand upon the helper is this: I must give up my power and my relationship—my will and my love—that others might live *their* lives more fully. Am I able to help?

We have returned to the point where we began in understanding response to human pain. The personal demands of the guts bring us back to the key, which is ourselves. Figure 6.1 shows the dialectic and the syntheses we have explored. The process moves between the taking in of what's there and the taking charge of what matters. These poles are distinguishable for the sake of analysis. They are partially separable in their activity. They intertwine in reality.

To respond is to be real. To be real is to ready *all* of oneself for what life calls forth. What matters most, in the end, is maintaining "an active, *thoughtful*" stance toward what is happening in life.[11] We are to be receptive actively, taking in the truth of situations. We are to be active receptively, shaping the meaning of situations. We are to live and respond in the faith which Kierkegaard described as floating in water 70,000 fathoms deep.[12]

Figure 6.1 The Pattern of Responding

Possibility	Predicaments	
	I am	I want
THE KEY	in everything	as everything
oneself		
Gestalt	ground	figure
THE CASE	pieces	parts
whole		
recognition of choices	shock of recognition	confrontation of intentions
THE GRAMMAR	caring	cognitive structure
healing	—special relationship	—rationale
	—special place	—procedures
approaches	evocative-insight oriented	directive-action oriented
STRESS	alarm	resistance
submission		
BRAIN	right hemisphere	left hemisphere
	—receptive	—active
	—nonrational	—rational
	—spatially oriented	—temporally oriented
	—intuitive	—intellectual
THE GUTS	experience	argument
knowledge		
Am I humble enough to respond?	Do I want to respond?	Am I tough enough to respond?

SPECIAL PAIN

Living includes dying,
and
death is the completion of living.
If health means wholeness,
and
wholeness includes the principles of
infirmity
and
death,
[then]
the healer
cannot adopt
a purely negative and hostile attitude
towards them.

Victor White [1]

7

Dependency

A drag! A martyr! A disaster!

This is the experience we have with a dependent personality. Every endeavor to relate seems thwarted. Every effort to respond comes to naught. Every attempt at ministry goes astray. One is bogged down, engulfed by the other's needs.

Let me put the problem differently: one does not know what the dependent person is experiencing. He or she withholds information necessary to the development of a mutually satisfying relationship. Thus one finds oneself doing extra work. The harder the responder tries to respond, the less satisfied the other seems. A little help mysteriously expands into the demand for a lot of helping. A little care somehow gets transformed into endless caring. What begins as meaningful support turns into an irritating albatross. One cannot figure out what has gone wrong.

The perplexity differs for those who are dependent. They experience themselves as dead, helpless, victimized, and so they behave as though they have no responsibility. Life does not depend on them. Something external determines the course of events. They themselves are unable to engage life in meaningful and significant ways.

But the perplexity of dependency is part of a total pattern of human interaction. The dependent personality is not a single pattern. There are varieties of dependent people, and their dependency is integrally intertwined with the patterns of others. Consequently, I will provide a larger cognitive map that puts together the variety of defensive-dependent patterns with those that are more responsively adaptive. This systematic picture can assist us in dealing more reflectively with the pain of human dependency.[2]

In presenting such a map of our transactions with each other, I am very aware that a map is not the territory, just as a menu does not constitute a meal. A map gives us some idea *about* the territory; a map provides no experience *of* the territory. A map aids us in developing a sense of what is covered and included. It is especially helpful when we are lost and need direction. On the other hand, when we know where we are going and are clear as to where we are, a map can be a nuisance.

A Larger Map

Certain assumptions underlie the map I will be using. Most of the time we take no notice of such assumptions, simply behaving as we do without an awareness of what is affecting our behavior. The value of making these assumptions explicit lies in the sharpened focus of the grammar—the structure—that shapes our responses to one another. Then we can change our responses in the light of our knowledge.

Most if not all that we do carries the intention of lessening our own discomfort. We act in such a way as to reduce anxiety. In short, our actions are directed. They are directed to create an interpersonal climate conducive to our sense of well-being.

Another closely related assumption is this: behavior is reciprocal. The assumption of interpersonal reciprocity is generally true, even though it may be inaccurate in specific instances. Behavioral responses tend to follow these sequences: dominance followed by submissiveness; submissiveness by dominance; hostility by hostility; and friendliness by friendliness. Robert Carson calls these reciprocal, high probability patterns "complementary." He argues that such interactions are reinforcing for both people because they maintain existing behavior patterns, reduce anxiety, and foster more relatedness. Contrariwise, conflicting patterns (i.e., dominance-dominance, submissiveness-submissiveness, hostile-friendly, and friendly-hostile interactions) generate more anxiety, do not reinforce behaviors, and increase the likelihood of the relationship ending. In other words, how we behave with each other is patterned with a high degree of probability but is not inevitable.

A shove usually provokes a countershove. A smile usually invites another's smile. Tears usually elicit tender sympathy. A request for help usually produces a helping response. Of course, these patterns do not always follow. Sometimes a shove is met with sympathy, a smile with a snarl, tears with anger, helplessness with thought-lessness. Then people become uncertain as to how to respond.

Another assumption is that all behavior is necessary in some form at some time. What we say and what we do are neither desirable nor undesirable in and of themselves. Everything depends upon the setting, the context, the situation in which they occur. Their degree of intensity, their quality of flexibility, their manifestation of balance and stability, and their fittingness all affect the way in which they are evaluated.

The assumption that all behavior may be fitting or ill-fitting, depending upon circumstances, underscores the conviction that there are times to be close and times to be distant, times to be assertive and times to be submissive, times to comfort and times to criticize.

Long ago the writer of Ecclesiastes (3:1-7, *The Jerusalem Bible*) poeticized the relativity of behavior: "There is a season for everything. . . . A time for tears, a time for laughter; a time for mourning, a time for dancing. . . . a time for embracing, a time to refrain from embracing. . . . a time for keeping silent, a time for speaking. . . ."

Another assumption undergirding the map I have constructed deals with the complexity of the human organism: namely, we are multileveled creatures. We are immediately aware of that complexity when we experience ourselves feeling one way inside and acting another way outside (see Romans 7:14-25).

There is the immediately apparent level of what everyone can see. This is *the public level*. It is available to others, though less available to oneself.

Similarly accessible is *the level of conscious intention*. Here I mean the experiences and reports of what one is thinking, feeling, and intending. It is made up of everything one says about oneself and one's world. It is deliberate.

Less easily accessible, though definitely present, is *the level of private symbolization*. Here we find dreams, fantasies, images, daydreams, and projections that provide the rich figurative, metaphorical, symbolic workings of the personality.

A fourth level is that of *conscience or valuation*. Here we deal with what matters to us: the ideas and convictions as to what is "good" and "right" and "real."

A further level reflects the farther reaches of humanity: *the ground of being itself*. Here is what matters ultimately, decisively, unreservedly: the source and center of life, that which brings us into being and calls us forth into our becoming.

When the pattern at each of these levels corresponds completely with the patterns of the other levels, there is a rigidity in the personality. Too little difference makes for a sterile sameness. Conflict is minimized and security maximized. Contrariwise, when the patterns are dramatically different, there is a chaos in the personality. Exaggerated difference makes for contradictory and competitive inconsistency, a convulsive civil war. Conflict is maximized and security minimized.

A final assumption, in preparation for the cognitive map of our interpersonal relationships, is that *people are different*. Even though, as human organisms, we possess the same basic stuff, we exhibit great variability.[3] The individual is always more than the species. The individual cannot avoid her or his individuality. What is helpful and desirable for one may not be so for another. We are different, and that difference makes a difference.

These, then, are five working assumptions about our patterns of interpersonal interaction:

1. we behave in order to reduce our own uncomfortableness;
2. our interaction with others is designed to elicit reciprocal responses that fit in with and continue behavior that reduces our anxiety;
3. how we behave may be adaptive or maladaptive, depending upon its frequency, balance, accuracy, and intensity;
4. personality exists on various levels, including the public and the conscious, which are interpersonal, and the private, the valuational, and the ground, which are intrapersonal;
5. despite a basic commonality, individuals are different in every respect.

With these assumptions before us, we can now turn to the map of our interactions with each other.

From a vast amount of both impressionistic material and empirical research, it is possible to chart what goes on between people in terms of a two-dimensional compass or diagram. That is, we can look at what goes on between us in terms of power or status which we either give to or take away from ourselves and others. Similarly, we can look at what goes on between us in terms of love or affiliation which we either move into or away from in relation to others.

Figure 7.1. The Interpersonal Relations Clock

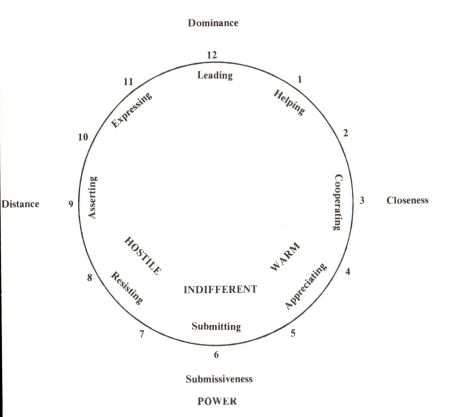

The power dimension may be thought of as a vertical dimension. It moves from a submissive stance at a position of 6 o'clock upward to a dominant stance at a position of 12 o'clock. In the power dimension, behaviors are intended to complement; that is, if one acts with dominance, one looks for a submissive response from the other. The love dimension may be thought of as a horizontal dimension. It moves from a close affiliative stance at 3 o'clock across to a distant and alone stance at 9 o'clock. In the love dimension, behaviors are intended to correspond; that is, if one acts hostilely, one looks for a hostile response from the other.

I use the points on the clock as a convenient, readily recognizable, and easy to remember diagram. However, the concept of the circle clock with specific points around it has deeper meaning.

In widely scattered cultures the circle has been a symbol of heaven and eternity and wholeness. Similarly, the square with its four axes has been a symbol of earth (with its four directions) and existence and time. Medieval philosophers tried mathematically to square the circle and to circle the square. They were seeking symbolically to reconcile heaven and earth, essence and existence, infinity and the finite. In the church, the closest approximation of heaven and earth coming together is the baptismal font, that is, the octagon, the eight-sided bowl, from which the waters of life are taken. So the circle clock with its hourly markers also indicates symbolic reconciliation of the whole of human interaction as well as a sharpening focus of the particulars of our interaction. With the circle we encompass everything at once; with the divisions we emphasize each thing in turn.

Think of the circle as a backboard with a half a court on either side, as shown in Figure 7.2.

If you throw a ball against the board from the right-hand side—12 o'clock through 3 o'clock to 6 o'clock—it will bounce back to that right side. In other words, a behavior initiated from the close affiliated side is intended to produce a close affiliated response. To return an intended close response with a distant one is to upset the other's security operation.

If you throw a ball against the board from the left-hand side—6 o'clock through 9 o'clock to 12 o'clock—it will bounce back to that left side. In short, a behavior initiated from the distant side is intended to produce a distant response. To return an intended distant response with a warm, friendly response is to disrupt the other's security pattern. This disruption is particularly baffling for most people in the helping professions. We are warm and friendly. When such responses only antagonize certain people, increasing their already uncomfortable pattern, we are bewildered. In fact, what is happening is our mistakenly moving too close at a time they are needing some distance.

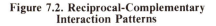
**Figure 7.2. Reciprocal-Complementary
Interaction Patterns**

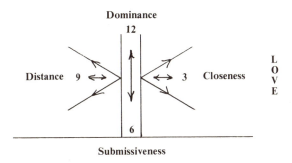

POWER

If you drop a ball from the top—12 o'clock straight down to 6
o'clock—or if you throw a ball up from the bottom—6 o'clock
straight up to 12 o'clock—it bounces neither to the close nor to the
distant side. Rather it stays in the more neutral middle.

In terms of the intensity pattern of behavior—fitting or ill-fitting
responses—if one throws the ball fast and hard against the wall, it will
hit and rebound with similar speed. On the other hand, if one gently
tosses the ball, it will rebound in a more manageable manner. Hard,
fast balls are difficult to handle. So, too, are intense, rigid behaviors.

Now let me go around the clock and designate more precisely the
power/love combinations at various points. The precise points are
too refined for our purposes, although careful research does this.
Instead, I am indicating about where they come on this interpersonal
compass:

11:30-1:00: *leadership patterns* of managing, directing, supervising

1:00-2:30: *helping patterns* of teaching, parenting, nurturing

2:30-4:00: *cooperative patterns* of nice, pleasant congeniality

4:00-5:30: *appreciative patterns* of responsiveness, respect,
teachableness

5:30-7:00: *submissive patterns* of dependency, obedience,
helplessness

7:00-8:30: *resistive patterns* of distrustfulness, skepticism,
powerlessness

8:30-10:00: *assertive patterns* of aggression, bluntness, anger

10:00-11:30: *expressive patterns* of calculation, competition, performance

A Sharper Focus

From this overall perspective, I will concentrate specifically on the dependency part of the compass. But since the dependent side assumes and requires the dominant side, we needed to see the interrelation of the two parts.

Fritz Perls referred to these two halves as the topdog/underdog patterns.[4] The topdog functions from a position of obvious power and high status, the upper half of the clock. The underdog functions from a position of low status and without obvious power, the lower half of the clock. The topdog tends to bully and browbeat. He or she manipulates with demands and threats. "If you don't do so-and-so, then you can expect to suffer such-and-such." The underdog tends to cower and cry. He or she manipulates with excuses and good intentions. "I really try, but I can't help it if things do not come out correctly." Whenever the conflict carries on over a period of time, the underdog always wins. The job never gets done. The task is never finished. The work is never correct. The topdog is frustrated. The underdog is blameless.

Three underdog patterns are identifiable:[5]
—the warmly dependent who appeals from a 4:00-5:30 position to strong supportive love in the 1:00-2:30 position;
—the indifferently dependent who appeals from a 5:30-7:00 position to strong leadership in the 11:30-1:00 position;
—the hostilely dependent who appeals from a 7:00-8:30 position to strong distance in the 10:00-11:30 position.

Each has similarities and differences. I will elaborate the patterns in turn and then draw together their common elements with some concrete directions for dealing with the drag of exaggerated dependency.

The Warmly Dependent Personality

The warmly dependent personality initially presents us with positive feelings. The person comes wanting to be friendly and close. Affiliation, identification, and proximity characterize the love dimension. What could be more desirable than the move to be together? That makes us feel good.

Similarly, the person comes acknowledging our strength and care. Appreciation, admiration, and teachableness characterize the power dimension. What could be more enhancing than the desire to receive from us? That makes us feel competent.

Remember, now, we are not dealing with normal, everyday give-and-take. We are focusing on exaggerated, too intense, inappropriate patterns of give-and-take. It is as if there are too many heavy towels and soaked sheets on one side of an automatic washer, causing it to stop its regular functioning. Let me describe this weighted behavior in more detail.

The compliant, warmly dependent person is saying something like this to us and to the world:

"I am unable really to take care of myself."

"I look to you to give me answers."

Such a person wants to remain the eternal child—taken care of forever. His or her behavior is intended to produce, elicit, and provoke from others tender, nurturing, and thoughtful instructing.

This person consequently suppresses, as do all underdogs, his or her own expansiveness and dominance. The substance of real living resides outside of oneself, so one always tries to please others. These others are invested with authority and so become the topdogs. In them is life, and that life might be available if only one is friendly and appreciative, close and submissive. One fears antagonism, for it could lead to the loss of support. That loss can be terrifying because one has denied in oneself and given to others the very qualities necessary for being itself.

By acting warmly dependent, one reduces the anxiety and uncomfortableness of having to be responsible. Behavior is directed toward getting from others the very support and strength one feels one does not have in oneself. Others experience the pull of caring, helping, nurturing, teaching and so tend to respond with strong, friendly behaviors. By pleasing and appeasing, one secures both protection and help. The behavior appeals to love.

The seeking of love from others, obviously, is neither unusual nor abnormal. It's love that "makes the world go round." However, the exaggerated seeking of strong love creates the drag of the warmly dependent personality.

There is a pattern of setting the other person up by a variety of strategies:

"If you love me, then you will not hurt me."

"I love you dearly; therefore, you should love me in return and give up everything for the sake of my love."

"Because you mean so much to me, you should take care of me and my needs."

"Since you are so wise and I admire your insight, you should share
your wisdom with me."

The personality, needs, and limitations of the strong, loving person
are disregarded. In part, that disregard is, as Karen Horney
characterized it, "a result of the anxiety which prompts the neurotic
to cling to the other person. One who is drowning and clings to a
swimmer does not usually consider the other's willingness or capacity
to carry him [or her] along."[6] All that matters is one's own
desperation at being left alone, deserted, and abandoned.

Precisely because one is both weak and warm, others are expected
to be strong and supportive.

The Indifferently Dependent Personality

The second underdog pattern takes on a somewhat different
configuration. As a person shifts the dominant locus of power-and-
love from the 4:00-5:30 area to the 5:30-7:00 area, we come upon a
more indifferently dependent personality. Rather than being either
warmly close or hostilely distant, the person tends to be neutral.
Nonchalance, detachment, and unconcern characterize the love
dimension. There is a kind of matter-of-factness in the relationship.
We are neither turned on nor turned off by such an individual.

Contrariwise, the person comes acknowledging our strength and
competence. Direction, domination, and leadership characterize the
power dimension. There is a strong expectation of our carrying the
full load of responsibility. We are built up and put on the spot by the
other.

The self-effacing, indifferently dependent person is saying
something like this to us and to the world:

"I can't handle what's here and I don't care what happens."

"You take charge because I will not."

"I am inadequate and inferior, so don't count on me."

Such a person wants to remain the eternal drifter—uninvolved
forever. His or her behavior is intended to produce, elicit, and
provoke strong leadership and direct domination.

This person is expressing his or her own exaggerated abasement.
One experiences oneself as nothing and so does not participate in
what goes on. Such an individual gives no evidence of expectations or
plans. "Who am I to want or need anything?" is the attitude. The
sense of resignation comes across powerfully and persuasively. What
one does grows increasingly limited. There is a restriction of wishes

and wants. No serious involvement can be seen. We feel the indifferently dependent to be an ever-present and an everlasting blob—a nonentity, a no-body, a nothing.

By acting nonchalantly dependent, one reduces the anxiety and uncomfortableness of having to be responsible and responsive in any way. That behavior is directed toward making others do what one feels (or is) unwilling to do oneself. Others experience the pull of managing, directing, bossing, domineering and so tend to respond with strong and impersonal behaviors. They are trained to look down on the indifferent person and to leave him or her alone. By apathy and resignation, one secures disengagement for oneself and more domination from the other. The withdrawal behavior is an appeal for freedom.

To seek freedom from others is neither unusual nor abnormal. In freedom we find breathing space necessary for our own being and becoming. But the exaggerated search to avoid real involvement creates the drag of the indifferently dependent personality.

There is a pattern of setting the other person up by a variety of strategies:

"Since you have the authority, you decide what to do."

"I really don't care what is done."

"It's up to you. I'll do whatever you say."

"Since I am a weak and inferior person, you must manage both of us."

Whatever initial direction we provide for such individuals quickly intensifies into chronic domination. We find ourselves irritated and annoyed by the lack of response. We disapprove of their behavior and eventually disregard their presence. By means of their compliant, resistant passivity, they successfully avoid outward activity and inward change. All that matters is getting out from under having to be part of anything and having to relate to anyone.

Precisely because one is both weak and withdrawn, others are expected to be strong and involved.

The Hostilely Dependent Personality

The third underdog pattern contrasts sharply with the other two. When someone responds out of a 7:00-8:30 position, he or she initially confronts us with negative feelings. The person stands away from us, wanting to be hostile and distant. Aloofness, lack of identification, and alienation characterize the love dimension. What could be more unsettling than a move against or apart from us. That makes us feel disliked and unloved.

Not dissimilarly, the person stands against us even as he or she acknowledges our power and strength. Resentment, cynicism, defiance, and bitterness characterize the power dimension. Our strength is conceded, but our stewardship of that power is questioned. We are set up and knocked down simultaneously. That makes us feel inadequate and unworthy.

The distrustful, hostilely dependent person is saying something like this to us and to the world:

"I know you are wrong, you S.O.B."

"You can't do anything right; you are always letting me down."

"Why do you always ignore my rights and overlook my needs?"

Such persons want to remain the everlasting brat—critically infantile forever. Their behavior is intended to produce, elicit, and provoke from others strong rejection and punishment.

These persons are expressing intense distrust. They experience themselves as victims, violated both by significant persons in their world and by the impersonal structures in which they find themselves. Others are blamed for their misery. Such persons are always throwing hand grenades into every situation. We can count on their criticism, their challenge of the commonly accepted and understood, and their complaints about the mishandling of every circumstance. Rather than seeking sympathy from us, they stress their grievances against us.

By acting defiantly dependent, one reduces the anxiety and uncomfortableness of having to be close and responsible. In other words, the hostilely dependent person does not want tender loving care. The expression of sullen disappointment is designed precisely to protect one against such responsiveness. As with a ball hurled against the backboard from a 7 o'clock position, the reaction sought is from an 11 o'clock position of strong rejection. The person is out to get the other to put him or her down while, at the same time, making the other feel attacked and undermined. The behavior is an appeal of anger.

The seeking of retaliation and distrust, obviously, is not usual. The exaggerated seeking of distant domination creates the drag of the hostilely dependent personality.

There is a pattern of setting the other person up by a variety of strategies:

"I have been disappointed and disillusioned by the world; there is nothing you can do for me."

"It is useless to collaborate because people cannot be trusted."

"I'm not like you and there's no way you could understand."

"The way things are done is wrong; everything you try only makes matters worse."

The personality, needs, and intentions of the dominant person are impugned and undermined. The individual delights in challenging what is generally accepted. He or she contests whatever comes along so intensely that there is little possibility for any kind of cooperation or collaboration. Because of the distantly critical cynicism, spontaneity and surprise are virtually eliminated from the relationship. All that matters is one's own protection against being close and responsible.

Precisely because one is both distrustful and defiant, others are expected to be unreliable and rejecting.

Core Qualities

Each pattern of dependency has its unique characteristics. The shift from the warmth of a 4 o'clock position to the coldness of an 8 o'clock position dramatizes these. At the same time, by virtue of the underdog position, all three patterns share common qualities. It is this commonality which I want to sharpen as a necessary step on the way to developing a strategy with which to cope with excessive dependency.

A basic passivity constitutes the most obvious common quality. The underdog refuses to assume responsibility for himself or herself. He or she participates in the interaction primarily to provoke others to take over and carry the load. One shows only enough cards to make others play the game. Overt effort is kept to a minimum. Deliberate avoidance is kept at a maximum. One's intentions are disguised and hidden. The person actively acts in ways designed to keep him or her from having to act. Because little that one does is out in the open, the individual experiences the loss of being an active agent in the world.

The loss of being an active person in the world produces a second fairly obvious common quality: namely, *the feeling of being a victim.* Because the person's intentions are disguised, others fail to meet

unvoiced expectations. That failure results in a continual source of disappointment and frustration for the dependent personality. His or her needs fail to be met in ways he or she wants them met:
"How could this [negative action] happen to me?"
"Why didn't you do this [positive action] for me?"
"How could you do this to me?"
Resentment and bitterness pervade the passivity and the dependency.

The dependent person feels that his or her own "good intentions" are all that count. Whether or not one invests oneself in the relationship is irrelevant. Whether or not one involves oneself in the task does not matter. All that counts is one's physical presence. One is there; what more could others want or expect!

Dependent people resent their dependency. Because of their need to please and to appear responsible, they disguise their resentment. They take part in activities hesitantly and reluctantly. They "forget" easily and often. They find "reasons" to slow things down. Behind a surface acquiescence lurks a deeper aggressiveness. "I will participate but I will withhold as much of myself as possible, for despite my dutifulness I have not been given what's due me." They resent going along, yet go along out of fear of losing the other or out of fear of having to be accountable. Not really knowing their own anxiety creates the experience of being a victim, they assume that the underdog status has been imposed by others.

A third core quality of dependent personalities is that *legitimate needs are transformed into* what Karen Horney spoke of as *neurotic claims*. What in fact is an understandable need gets changed into a special, exceptional, inalienable right.

"I need to be taken care of; others, therefore, must take care of me."
"The world should be at my service and I should not be bothered."
Things ought to come without one having to make an effort.

Unconditional care and concern are expected regardless of one's own provocative behavior. No matter how one acts, one deserves the best. No matter what the circumstances, one's needs are to be met then and there without delay. Simply because one desires help, one deserves help. The world exists for one's own purposes.

The suffering of dependent personalities works to bolster the legitimacy of their claims. The difficulties they meet in trying to please others make them special. The handicaps they labor under in trying to make it in life prove they are exceptional. By means of misery, they manage to accuse others of failure and at the same time to excuse themselves of their own failure. Suffering sears others and salves themselves.

A Nasrudin story illustrates the inadequacies of the conventional view of life, especially as regards who gets taken when ordinary needs turn into extraordinary claims. One day the Mulla was walking along an alley when a man fell off a roof and landed on top of him. The victim was unhurt, but Nasrudin had to be taken to the hospital. When asked by his disciples what teaching he inferred from the event, he exclaimed: "Avoid belief in inevitability, even if cause and effect seem inevitable! Shun theoretical questions like: 'If a man falls off a roof, will his neck be broken?' *He* fell—but *my* neck is broken!"[7]

The underdog always manages to come out on top. The topdog invariably ends up on the bottom. The intense vindictive reaction to the frustration of claims—"How can they do this to me?"—results in an assault upon others. With the warmly dependent person, others are made to feel guilty for not nurturing. With the indifferently dependent person, others are made to feel a failure for not leading. With the hostilely dependent person, others are made to experience blame for not performing. The problem ends up being that of the strong others, while the weak one is never in the wrong.

What one needs gets exaggerated into what one deserves. What one deserves becomes translated into one's rightful claim without conditions and without qualifications:

love from others . . .

freedom for oneself . . .

anger against others. . . .

These are dependent persons' inalienable rights. No questions can be asked. No quarter can be given. These are theirs regardless. So runs their inner logic. *They* fall, but *our* necks are broken.

Directions for Coping

I confess that I have not found any easy way to manage the drag of dependency. However, this analysis of the patterns of love and the positions of power has provided me with some directions for dealing with excessive dependency. I present these as suggestions. I hope that they will provide clues for discerning what goes on between you and others and provide alternatives for managing the frustrations.

I put the basic issue in the form of a question: *who does what work in the relationship?*

Martin Luther stressed the fact that nobody can perform the most basic human acts for another. Nobody can believe for me; nobody can be baptized for me; nobody can die for me. These—and other—fundamental personal acts can only be done by myself. There can be no proxies, no stand-ins, no substitutes. Either I respond or there is no response. Either I work or there is no work accomplished. Either I grow or there is no growth in me. Meaning for myself is my work, work which nobody else can do on my behalf.

As a strong and supportive helper or a strong and involved leader or a distrusted and rejecting exploiter (depending upon the pattern of the dependent person), I can advance ideas, hunches, strategies, meanings. They are all grist for the mill. But in the end—in that decisive moment of transformation from the possible to the actual—it is the other who thinks and knows and acts. And if the other does not, no thinking and no knowing and no acting on my part matters.

What works for us may or may not work for others. This is especially so when we experience the pressure of the dependent person to have us do his or her work. My meaning, the way I connect this event with that event, can never finally constitute another's meaning, the way the other connects this event with that event. I can provide ingredients—the grammar of a responding relationship—yet I can never produce the completed course. Each one must do that for oneself.

So, whenever you experience the undertow, the drag of dependency in another, examine closely who is doing what work in the relationship. Whenever you find you are feeling too supportive or too directive or too exploitative, you may be certain you have taken over too large a share of the load. Even more, under such circumstances you are doing what you can not do: namely, express the uniqueness of another's life experience. Each person, observes Paul, has one's own proper burden of being to bear (see Galatians 6:5, NEB).

The initial issue of "who does what work" seeks to clarify what is mine and what is not mine in the responding relationship. A second issue deals with my active responding: *how can I interrupt the destructive dependency?*

Because of the exaggerated intensity of the dependent responses, we may find ourselves provoked into reacting in certain ways. We feel an obligation to care about the other. We know the demand to dominate the other. We sense the pressure to exploit the other. We find ourselves trapped in a box of logical illogicalness. The harder the ball of behavior is thrown at us and the closer to the edge of the circle of responses it originates, the more difficult to stop or deflect it. The dependent person narrows his or her actions in such an aggressive way that the world around is trained to take over.

It is that pattern of setting others up to take over that we must interrupt and dislodge. Thus, if the hostilely dependent person comes across from an intense 8 o'clock position, bitterly angry and accusatively critical, an appropriate way to sidestep the attack and to right the balance is to ask: "How would you handle it?" "What suggestions do you have that can help?" In other words, we respond from a position of strength that prods the other's response without rejecting or destroying the other. The attitude tends toward passive friendliness, cool but not cold, calm without clobbering. The corresponding and complementary responses are maintained but without the dysfunctional intensity which had been sought in the dependency. One is distant and dominant appropriately.

Or, if the indifferently dependent person pulls back from an intense 6 o'clock position, withdrawn and whining, an appropriate way to sidestep the opting-out-capitulation and to right the balance is to declare: "Since it does not matter to you, it will be done this way." "Since you want out, it will go on without you." In other words, we respond from a position of strength that frees the other without dominating or destroying the other. The attitude tends toward the matter-of-fact: "This is it—do what you want, I can't change the way things are." The corresponding and complementary responses are maintained but without the desired maladaptive intensity. One is neutral and directive appropriately.

Or, if the warmly dependent person comes on from an intense 4 o'clock position, close and clinging, an appropriate way to sidestep the hanging-on parasite and to right the balance is to encourage: "I'm not certain about this, what ideas do you have that we might try?" "Come on, put your mind to work; you've got good ideas when you give yourself a chance; what kinds of things come to mind?" In other words, we respond from a position of strong support that inspires the other without belittling or browbeating him or her. The attitude tends toward active friendliness, reaching out without taking over, close without smothering. The corresponding and complementary responses are maintained but without their exaggerations. One is friendly and supportive appropriately.

The dependent person comes on as an underdog yet invariably

ends up on top. Those who appeared to be victors find themselves victims. And those who looked like victims turn out to be victors. The difficulty in such reversal, however, comes with the realization that every victor/victim relationship constitutes a loss for *every*one. To interrupt disruptive behavior is to modify the direction of the interaction from the irresponsible toward the responsible.

Once clear about *who* does what work, the next step is to recognize *how* to assist the other to do his or her work. That requires a strong effort to stop the powerful drive for dominance on the part of the person in the overtly underdog position and to start the slow redirection toward a more satisfying reciprocity.

A third issue is implicit in my actively responding to interrupt the destructive dependency. That is: *how can I convey to the other some sense of his or her significance?*

Most of us struggle with feelings of uncertainty about ourselves. Much of the time these are not intense; occasionally, they rise like a flood, threatening to drown us in the waters of worthlessness. Usually, such feelings are minor in intensity and manageable in their effects.

For despotically dependent persons, however, the sense of insignificance ruthlessly rules their lives. These people not only feel, but also believe, that they can have no real say in their lives. Their position does not warrant it; their abilities to cope do not include it.

"You are the one who can do it," is the admiring response of the warmly dependent.
"I cannot do it, you have to," is the submissive response of the indifferently dependent.
"Why can't you do it right," is the critical response of the hostilely dependent.

In all cases, the underdog discloses personal feelings of inability *and* of insignificance.

Our task is to transform that "I can't" into an "I won't" at least or into an "I will" at best. We have to find ways to aid the dependent person to move from a feeling that he or she can have no say to a feeling that he or she has some say. To get a person to assert "I won't do this" instead of settling for "I can't do this" is to enable one to be responsible for not acting responsibly. At the core of unhealthy powerlessness lies a healthy power. It is that power—that source of ability and intention, that source of significance and satisfaction— which we seek to liberate.

No one can give another a sense of significance. All we can do is to resist the undertow of helplessness and hopelessness. All we can do is to encourage the flowing tide of risking responsiveness. We shift the focus from ourselves to the other, from our carrying the weight of the other's life to the other carrying the weight of his or her own life. As the balance of burden shifts to a proper balancing of interdependency, what had once been a drag turns into a source of delight.

We seek to pull behavior patterns away from the lopsided outer ring of the behavioral circle and to move them closer toward the functioning center. We find, in the end, that all of us have times when we need and want to be close and taken care of by others. We appeal to love from others. We all have times when we need and want to be left alone and not bothered by others. We appeal to freedom for ourselves. We all have times when we need and want to be critical and skeptical about what is going on. We appeal to proper anger against what is happening. Such balancing fosters more fully functioning persons.

In our day a martyr has come to mean the masochistically dependent person. Such a person allows others to do him or her in in debilitating and destructive ways. So we speak of the "martyr complex."

Originally, in the time of the early church, however, martyr meant the opposite. A martyr was one who showed forth—who declared—who witnessed to—the living, vital faith that sustained his or her life. It is that freedom of being-in-the-world-for-the-sake-of-all which we seek for others *and* for ourselves.

8

Aging

A ninety-two-year-old woman lay in bed in her daughter's home. In preceding months, her life had grown deeply disturbing: unrelieved agony, constant confusion, the indignity of utter helplessness, and the aggravation of aggressive concern on her part to be self-sufficient canceled by her inability to be trusted to take care of anything. In an especially poignant episode, her daughter found her crawling around the bed agitatedly searching among the covers. When asked what she wanted, she replied, "I'm looking for my lost self."

The haunting fear of aging turns into a full-blown nightmare in senility. Even if one does not become a vegetable, one knows one is not oneself. Like that ninety-two-year-old, even in that pathetic condition of having lost one's centeredness, one is enough oneself to realize that one is not oneself.

Aging is a reality that comes to all. It represents the accumulated continuity of time and living. Though aging comes to all, it is not the same for all. It is subtle, varied, mixed. Senility is a reality that comes to some. It symbolizes the most exaggerated pain of the oldness that can come with aging. It is all too obvious, all too limiting, all too tragically pathetic. To be aged is to have to face the prospect of possibly being senile.

Until recently, aging loomed as forbodingly as death. A conspiracy of silence iron-curtained the elderly, the infirmed, the senile. As outcasts, old people have been "condemned to poverty, decrepitude, wretchedness and despair." [1]

Age now divides people into "good" versus "bad" as ruthlessly as race and sex have. Agism has been added to racism and sexism.

I propose to look at the *human* pain of aging from within the phenomenon itself, as people have experienced it. Next, I will put those reflections into more abstract statements. Then I will explore some directions for meeting whatever we must or might meet in terms of aging.

Experience from Within

While age takes us by surprise, as Goethe observed,[2] many find themselves looking for the signs of its appearing. Like adolescent preoccupation with the body, as we move into "the middle ages" we scan our features in the mirror looking for evidence of gray hair and wrinkles around the eyes, or we gaze at our hands and forearms looking for the rippled surface and the blotchy skin. That which will not happen to us, one day does happen to us and continues to happen to us. We are aging!

Intense feelings of fleeting age produce a frozen past, a limited future, and a crushing present. One finds less and less space, more and more constriction, fewer and fewer resources, more and more darkness; yet all the while one continues to experience oneself as being the same person. There is the baffling question, "Can I have become a different person while I am still myself?"

As a way of getting into the experience more fully, try the following:

Get comfortable and close your eyes. Imagine you are in a large room. The room is filled with many objects—furniture, pictures, books, sculpture, knick-knacks, vases, and so on—that reflect and express who you are. Move about the room. Go where you like. Do what you like. Examine the objects. Attend to those that you cherish especially. Rearrange the room, if you like.

Now you see something on the far side of the room that you want. You start across to get it; suddenly you slam into a glass wall. The glass is so clear that you had not seen it. You pick yourself up and continue enjoying your room. Only now, while you can still see your room, you can no longer move around as much as you had. . . .

Again you see something you want to investigate. Again you start over to it. Again you slam into a glass wall, invisible but solid.

Now the glass walls are becoming cloudy. You can no longer see as clearly. You cannot move as freely. You still cherish your room. You can still rearrange part of it, but space is smaller and objects fewer.

Suddenly, your room turns into a horror movie nightmare. There are cloudy glass walls on every side, moving in and in and in, closer and closer and closer. Stay with the experience. Let the feelings flood through you. What thoughts race through your head? What do you try to do? What is happening?

Now in your imagination come back to the room and the chair where you are. Open your eyes and look around.

With the experience of aging, an open life imperceptibly merges into a limited life. Whereas there is a time when there are few if any boundaries, there comes a time when there is nothing but boundaries. Abilities go; memory decays; what one has worked so hard to create is labor lost; the end is as though there had been no beginning. Even so, however limited and exiled in the present, the old person still remains the person he or she was.

Like lepers in olden times, the old feel what it means to be untouchable outcasts! As in the Persian proverb, the old find that instead of being on the saddle, the saddle is now on them.[3] The experience is seldom, if ever, pleasant. It comes as a surprise, though inevitable. It brings limitations and liabilities, loneliness and loss.

Analysis from Without

Turn now to a more objective analysis of aging. Temporarily set aside personal poignancy for the sake of descriptive understanding.

Clearly, aging is a developmental process within the limits of finitude. We are born, we grow, we mature, we decline, we die. Like a trajectory there is an initial blast-off, an arching height, and a final descent. More precisely, aging focuses upon the later stages of the life cycle.

These later stages may be divided into three unequal yet

distinguishable phases: the middle years, later maturity, and old age.[4]

The middle years are, in truth, just that: the mid-period between an unformed beginning and a fairly fixed ending. Here is a plateau, beginning around thirty-five and extending into the early sixties. Under normal circumstances there are few gross changes in our behavior, in our attitudes, or in our activities. We experience some decline in energy. We become more sensitive to the rush of time. Years accumulate with increasing rapidity. In contrast to physical activity, we tend to look more to mental activity for satisfaction and recognition. Even though there is occasional tiredness, life remains full, active, intact.

Sometime in the mid-sixties, our life pattern shows more noticeable changes. This is the period of *later maturity*. We experience increasing difficulty with extensive involvements. Coping with life's exigencies requires more coping skill. We experience fewer assets and more deficiencies. Losses begin to exceed gains. It is harder to keep life together; we can do it, but only with a greater expenditure of energy. The speed of the car shifts from third to second gear.

Finally, for some there comes that period to which the greatest anxiety is related: namely, *old age*. It may come in the late sixties. It is more likely to come in the late seventies for some, not until the late eighties for others, and not until the early nineties for a few. We slam into extreme limitations. Life is decisively constricted and even disorganized. We are fragile, perhaps disabled, and virtually done in. At best we merely manage to exist. At worst we simply vegetate. The nightmare of aging turns into the trauma of senility.

Senility as the frightening face of aging conveys the greatest threat of all:[5] long-term chronic illness, institutionalization, loss of independent status. When we no longer have a sense of dignity and when we no longer possess a sense of self-determination, then we no longer are ourselves. A terrifying Other has taken over our reliable self. We are lost, yet *we* continue to live on.

Through the years theories as to what constitutes successful aging have varied.[6] Basically, there are two: activity and disengagement. Recent research, however, suggests that these are oversimplifications. On the one hand, it is important to maintain a certain level of activity. On the other, it is desirable to draw together the varied strands of one's life.

Evidence supporting both the activity *and* disengagement theories (instead of either/or) appeared in the Kansas City Study on Aging.[7]

Researchers examined (*i*) personality types, (*ii*) role activities, and (*iii*) life satisfactions of several hundred people between the ages of fifty and eighty over a six-year period. Role activity meant the extent and intensity of a person's involvement in twelve different roles: parent, spouse, grandparent, kin, group member, worker, homemaker, citizen, friend, neighbor, club and association member, and church member. Life satisfaction included pleasure in daily activities, life being meaningfully met, successful goal accomplishment, positive self-image, and happy and optimistic attitudes and moods. On the basis of comparing role activities and life satisfactions, they developed a pattern of personality types which are elaborated below.

The sample includes "only those relatively advantaged 70-year-olds who have better-than-average health, cooperativeness, and general well-being." This very skewing obscures the more ravaging effects upon older persons wrought by the injustices of our socioeconomic system. For those who have, the last may not be too bad; for those who have not, the last is worse than ever.

Within each of the four major personality types, the researchers established further divisions according to the level of role activity and according to life-satisfaction ratings. Table 8.1 shows the four types—the "integrated," the "defended," the "passive-dependent," and the "disintegrated" or "unintegrated"—as well as the subtypes.

The *"integrated"* personality type represents the optimum. The person functions well. He or she has a complex inner life. One is intact intellectually and is competent personally. There is a flexibleness, a mellowness, a maturity that characterizes one's activities and satisfactions. Within the "integrated" type are three distinguishable subtypes. There is the "reorganizer" who competently enjoys a broad range of activities. He or she stays young, remains active, finds substitute involvement as limitations appear, and refuses to grow old. The "focused" subtype reduces the range of involvement by a self-conscious selectivity and prioritizing. The third subtype, the "disengaged," is that person who exhibits calm contentment with a deliberate decision to withdraw from active involvement. He or she displays a "rocking-chair" approach to a peaceful life.

The second main personality type is called the *"armored"* or *"defended"* type. These individuals disclose a pattern of ambitious striving for achievement. They maintain a tight control over their impulse life to defend against anxiety. Within this type are two

Table 8.1
Personality Type in Relation to Activity and Life Satisfaction (Age 70-79)
(N=59)

Personality Type	Role Activity	Life Satisfaction High	Medium	Low
Integrated	High	9 A	2	
	Medium	5 B		
	Low	3 C		
Armored-Defended	High	5 D		
	Medium	6	1	
	Low	2	1 E	1
Passive-Dependent	High		1 F	
	Medium	1	4	
	Low	2	3	2 G
Unintegrated	High		2	1
	Medium	1		
	Low		2	5 H
	Total	34	16	9

Name of Pattern

A—Reorganizer	E—Constricted
B—Focused	F—Succorance Seeker
C—Disengaged	G—Apathetic
D—Holding On	H—Disorganized

From Bernice L. Neugarten, Robert F. Havighurst, and Sheldon S. Tobin. In Bernice L. Neugarten, ed., *Middle Age and Aging: A Reader in Social Psychology* (Chicago: University of Chicago Press, 1968), p. 174. Diagram reprinted by permission of the University of Chicago Press.

subtypes. First, there are those who "hold on" as long and as fully as possible to the involvements of middle age under the threats of aging. Second are the "constricted." They are preoccupied with the threat of loss and limitation. They reduce their involvements and endeavor to close themselves off from experience. They pull out rather than hang in.

Two patterns emerge among the *"passive-dependent"* types. There is the "succorance-seeking" group who constantly seek a responsiveness from others for their strong dependency needs. As long as they can find someone to take care of these needs, they can maintain themselves fairly well. The other subgroup is "apathetic." They tend to be "rocking-chair" people but with a much different character structure. These people reveal low activity and low satisfaction. The aging process reinforces engrained patterns of passivity and apathy. Nothing matters and nothing satisfies. They display the indifferently and hostilely dependent patterns described in the previous chapter— but exaggerated by aging.

The final personality type is the *"unintegrated"* or *"disorganized."* Here we find gross psychological defects, loss of emotional control, and deterioration of thought processes.

The researchers suggest that there is no sharp discontinuity between the young and the old. We become, perhaps even more, what we have always been. With age there comes an increasing consistency of personality type. An individual "impresses" his or her own style upon the changes that occur. One "ages according to a pattern that has a long history and that maintains itself, with adaptation, to the end of life."

I have described some of the experience of aging from the inside. I have also reported some analysis of the process from an objective viewpoint. Now I intend to deal more specifically with directions for responding to the human pain of aging.

What can we do to reduce the painfulness and to enhance the meaningfulness of aging? What can optimize its assets? What can minimize its liabilities?

Directions

The underlying assumptions as to what constitutes meaningful aging are the same as those of meaningful living at any age. They are not age-specific. Instead they are ageless. They apply to all.

Maggie Kuhn, leader of the Gray Panthers, a national organization of militant old people fighting for "a non-bingo way of life" for the elderly, has outlined the needs of older people in such a way as to underscore the agelessness of *human* need.[8] There are four such needs:

—awareness of oneself and one's identity as a responsible person;
—confidence in one's own experience;
—involvement in decision-making processes;
—transcendent interests reflecting meaning and significance in living.

I will say more about the Gray Panthers later, but for now this articulation of the needs of older people shows the continuity with the needs of younger people. Despite obvious, conspicuous, and monumental differences, we are more alike than we are different.

Transition marks the sharpness of the aging process. Yet transition characterizes every age: from the womb to the world; from the home to the school; from the school to the world of work; from living with one's natural family to living in one's acquired family; from seeking to become settled to having settled in; from many involvements to fewer involvements; from middle age to later maturity to old age. Transition—anticipated, remembered, known, experienced, feared—distinguishes events from the ongoing. The awareness of change symbolizes our peculiarly human predicament.

Under conditions of change we are forced to reorient ourselves in terms of time and space. Much of the difficulty older people experience in moving from their "home" into "a smaller place" is not simply the thankless and poignant task of deciding about the accumulated possessions of the years. That decision-making is hard enough: What do we do with these letters? What about those photographs? Can we throw out these certificates of recognition? What are we to do with the children's baby things? And so the process goes. Almost every object reawakens long forgotten yet living memories, memories that remind us of who we are. But more than the throwing out is the uncertainty of the projected moving in. We have to reorient ourselves to find another "place." We have to reorganize our "possessions" in order to dwell in the land of the living. And that takes a mobilization of all the energy we have plus a good deal more!

For older people transitions tend to be especially traumatic. One moves from a known life space in which there is breathing room into an unknown constricted space where there may not be room to roam. It is that collapsing of space that lies within the terrible prospect of senility. In its less acute form, the trauma of transition finds expression in the anticipation of institutionalization. One sees oneself inevitably driven from relative autonomy into residential care.

Because of the focal fear of institutionalization and its corollary anxiety of confused old age, let's look more closely at strategies to lessen the aggravation of aging. I have learned these through serving as a clinical consultant to a home for the elderly, meeting with the staff about patients and residents who have been difficult to understand and to help.

Basic approaches to the confused elderly person are known as Reality Orientation and Attitude Therapy.[9] They are widely used in geriatric settings. They assume that individuals can be helped by a coherent and consistent treatment program based upon an understanding of the individual's behavior problems and patterns.

Reality Orientation is a retraining program aimed at the confusion stemming from severe organic cerebral deficiency. The individual is no longer able to keep facts straight. There is a loss of dignity and self-determination. Attention span is short and confusion great. With a careful program of relearning one's name—recovery of one's basic identity—and of offering simple information as to time, place, and activity, the person becomes reoriented to reality. In a friendly, calm, direct, and slow atmosphere, the person engages in simple, familiar, and persistent activities. The repetitive consistency literally works wonders whenever confusion is present and one's usual controls are undermined.

In contrast to, although in combination with, Reality Orientation, Attitude Therapy deals with the interpersonal exchanges between individuals. It is a carefully planned attitude approach to treatment that endeavors to decrease and extinguish undesirable behaviors and to increase and reinforce desirable behaviors. It requires consistency on the part of everyone who has contact with the patient or resident. It is maintained around the clock. Like young children, old people do not have the adaptability and flexibility to cope easily with inconsistency in the environment. When individuals vary in the way they deal with the person, therefore, confusion, frustration, uncertainty, anxiety, aggravation, irritation, and rage follow. The less the consistency, the greater the resulting upset. The greater the consistency, the less the resulting upset.

The prescribed attitudes represent elementary interpersonal concepts. Supposedly they are simple to teach and easy to learn. I say "supposedly" because prior to my consultation relationship St. Ann's had been conscientiously applying Reality Orientation and Attitude Therapy for two years with discouraging results. They understood and applied the attitudes in somewhat mechanical ways. My consultation introduced a fuller view of interpersonal behavior with a resulting improvement in the success of the program. But the scaffolding of prescribed attitudes based on identifiable behavior patterns constitutes the heart of the approach.

There are five attitudes in all. Each is used according to an understanding of the patient's or resident's behavior. In many instances, more than one attitude is followed. After describing the attitudes, I will report on an evaluation of the approach so you can sense something of its usefulness.

Active Friendliness (AF) is used with the shy, withdrawn person. Such an individual feels little worth and little adequacy. Self-confidence is low and diffidence is high. He or she is given much personal support and structure for successful experience. One takes the initiative in extending attentiveness before the individual requests it. "Your hair ribbon looks so lovely today." "Mr. Jones, here's a shoelace. I noticed you need one." "What is that you are doing? It looks very interesting." The approach is not a matter of making something up, for that is really being disrespectful and manipulative. Rather, it is finding something in the person's situation that one can respond to and reinforce genuinely. One takes the initiative for the involvement.

Passive Friendliness (PF) is used with the suspicious and apprehensive person. Such an individual feels uncomfortable with and fears too much closeness and too much warmth. The world is not to be trusted. One is available and alert to this personality type yet lets him or her make the first response. The person is allowed to move at his or her own pace. One is courteous but not companionable. One says "hello" but does not engage in conversation. One maintains contact but at a distance. One lets the other have the initiative for whatever involvement there is.

Matter-of-Factness (MF) is used whenever a person attempts to manipulate or control the environment for self-defeating and/or disruptive purposes. He or she may complain constantly about bodily difficulties or the regular routine. The pattern is designed to elicit sympathy on the one hand and to get out from under responsibility for his or her behavior on the other. The attitude to be used is a limit-setting, straight-forward "this is the way things are" approach that undercuts a power struggle, tug-of-war between the other and oneself. One affirms but does not justify. One insists but does not condemn. Without being diverted by arguments and complaints, one keeps control over decisions and directions.

Kind Firmness (KF) sounds similar to Matter-of-Factness yet is significantly different. It is the most difficult of the attitudes for people to understand and to implement. It is intended for the person whose anger and hostility are directed inward instead of outward— the depressed individual. To praise or encourage a person in such a condition only makes him or her feel worse. The trick is to get the person working at a menial, monotonous, and unsatisfying task. One neither encourages nor praises. All that matters is that the job be done. One keeps the person involved in the deadly drudgery, kindly but without sympathy, firmly but without punishing. Eventually, the person's anger turns outward—against the situation, against the taskmaster, against the injustice. Once the person "blows up," the depression lifts and more normal interaction can occur.

The final attitude is No Demand (ND) and is used with the individual under conditions of uncontrollable and generalized rage. Such a person is hostile and threatening, attempting to frighten others away by the vehemenace of reaction. One backs off in such a situation, waiting for the storm to subside. Other activities and concerns are offered but not pressed. A power struggle, either verbal or physical, is avoided. To attempt to reason with the person in an unreasonable rage only aggravates the situation. One isolates and protects and waits. After the person has quieted down, one can explain what is and is not helpful, how the program is set up, and what can and cannot be done. The only demands in the midst of an eruption are protective; preventing harm to the person himself or herself and harm to others. Otherwise, one avoids every demand upon the person to do anything at that time.

Each of these attitude approaches can be understood as part of the more systematic analysis of interpersonal interaction presented in the chapter on dependency. Active Friendliness represents a response from about a 2 o'clock position to an appeal to love from about a 4 o'clock position. (See Figure 8.3.) It is intended to elicit warm dependency and increasing self-confidence. Matter-of-Factness represents a response from about a 12 o'clock position to an appeal to direction and control from about a 6 o'clock position. It is intended to

Table 8.2. Attitudes and Behaviors

ATTITUDE	BEHAVIOR PATTERN	PRESCRIBED ACTION
(AF) Active Friendliness	Withdrawn, apathetic, diffident	Initiating warm contact
(PF) Passive Friendliness	Suspicious, apprehensive	Waiting for other's responsiveness
(MF) Matter-of-Factness	Manipulative, complaining, demanding	Setting limits
(KF) Kind Firmness	Depression	Enforcing aggravating drudgery
(ND) No Demand	Out of control	Eliminating demands

Table 8.2 sets out the five attitudes and their prescribed patterns.

Figure 8.3. Attitudes and the Interpersonal
Relations Clock

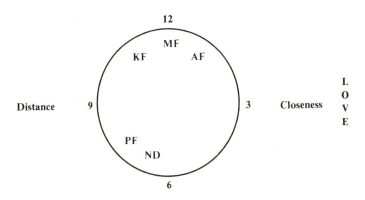

AF Active Friendliness
KF Kind Firmness
MF Matter-of-Factness
ND No Demand
PF Passive Friendliness

elicit an uncomplaining obedience. Kind Firmness represents a response from about a 10:30 position to an appeal to anger from about an 8:30 position. It is intended to elicit an openly hostile dependence. No Demand represents a response from about 6:30 to an appeal for freedom from obligations from about an 11:30 position. It is intended to elicit control and direction. Passive Friendliness represents a response from about 7 o'clock to an appeal for distance from about an 11 o'clock position. It is intended to elicit assertion and initiative.

Most of us in the helping professions are doing what we do because we want to help others. We come at our jobs from the right side of the circle clock, namely, a response of friendly identification. But you will notice that Matter-of-Factness, Kind Firmness, Passive Friendliness, and No Demand each reflect a response of some distance. There is an otherness, an over-againstness, an objectivity to these. This does not mean that the responses are far out on the edge of the circle, for that would mean, you remember, exaggerated and maladaptive behavior. Rather this means the responses are located slightly distant—MF, KF, PF, ND—and either more powerful—MF, KF—or less powerful—PF, ND.

At the end of the first year and a quarter of the consultation, we evaluated what had happened. We sought to assess whether the patients/residents had improved, not changed, or gotten worse as a result of the treatment program. "Improvement" meant the staff felt more able to cope with the person and felt less undermined and discouraged by what was happening. "Worse" meant the staff felt less able to cope and more undermined and discouraged.

The percentage of people not changing or getting worse seems to stabilize around 15 percent. Rather remarkably, about 85 percent of those who initially were causing enough disturbance to require special attention improved.

A closer examination of the attitudes used aids an understanding of who improves and who does not. Fewer than a quarter had an Active Friendliness prescribed. Almost half required Matter-of-Factness. Many required a combination of attitudes as the person exhibited changes in behavior. For example, Matter-of-Factness would be used with an impulsive or manipulative response, while No Demand would be called upon when agitation and upset got too much. The greatest difficulties, based upon a statistical reading, come with individuals who require a combination of Passive Friendliness for their suspiciousness and fear of closeness and of No Demand for their uncontrollable rage.

The crux of the issue of direction in responding to the *human* pain of aging revolves around the matter of one's identity and sense of integrity. These are concepts which Erik Erikson has given prominence. One's identity points to "a persistent sense of sameness within oneself (selfsameness) and a persistent sharing of some kind of essential character with others."[10] In other words, I have a sense of myself as myself; I have a sense of fostering and encouraging that same self over time; others recognize a continuity over time of who I appear to be to them; there is a large overlap between who I see myself to be and who others see me as being. One's integrity points to an emotional acceptance and integration of one's own and only life cycle and style of life.[11] One feels at home in the person one is. One can view with respect the character of one's life.

We are to encourage and enhance such identity and integrity. How? By providing experiences and activities in which people can be involved in a variety of roles.[12] That requires flexibility: being a friend, being a helper, being a grandparent, being a church member, being a neighbor, and so on. Within these various roles there needs to be an element of giving and not simply receiving.

Earlier I alluded to the Gray Panthers. They are providing a model for a different life-style, especially in later maturity. It is a life-style of independence and outrage. Old age brings more than its share of rage, frustration at the indignities and infirmities of the senile process. It behooves us to remember the root of anger underneath the upset of the elderly. The Gray Panthers seek to turn outrage into action as well as service.

People in later maturity, contends Maggie Kuhn, at last are free enough from obligations to "rattle the cages." They can mobilize the resources of a lifetime of experience to fight against "those things that diminish and oppress" us all. Thus, they draw upon the varied backgrounds of the retired to tackle problems in transportation, health, maintenance, banking, tax reform, and the courts. With enforced leisure there looms the potent consolidation of wisdom *and* advocacy. "God might just use the people who are nearest to death," she asserts, "to point to new life."[13]

While I have been focusing on the preliminary fear of aging and the ultimate anxiety of senility, all that I have been writing in this chapter is only a variation on all *human* pain. The tragedy of old age is but a mirror reflection of the tragedy of every age. That was brought home to me with powerful and poignant impact one day.

I had visited an eighty-two-year-old woman and her husband over a period of months. She was bedridden, living out the slow workings of death by cancer. A demanding person, she always complained about never getting enough of anything. Consequently, I confess I did not look forward to our visits and performed them reluctantly.

One particular day, after we had read some Scripture and prayed together, I rose to go. Only this time she seemed to me a different person. Her face looked serene and beautiful. On impulse, I bent over and kissed her on the cheek. She startled—and humbled—me with her response.

"Why I'm not ugly after all. I'm not ugly after all."

Perhaps that is what human pain is all about. Are we ugly or lovely? Can we give love and receive love even to our life's end?

9

Dying

Loving and living go together (see 1 John 3:14). When one is not lovable and loving, then one experiences a living death. So the pain of lonely unlovableness haunts us as the most excruciating pain of all and the warmth of a caring love heals most human pain.

While most people fear the process of aging with its projected fear of indignity, it is the process of dying with its projected years of extreme dependency and excruciating pain that looms as the final obstacle to meaningful living. For those who have seriously avoided facing life, facing death comes as a cruel execution. For those who have found a sense of self and integrity with who one is and what one has done, facing death comes as a calm experience to be met and mastered as have previous experiences.

Regardless of the contrast between those who flee from life and those who face life, dying is not a casual experience nor is death an ordinary event. Dying confronts us with the issue of the means of living—maintaining a sense of dignity. Death faces us with the issue of the meaning of life—finding purpose in the presence of the unknown. Both confront us with intensification of *human* pain.

In the midst of our everyday routine, this intensification can be easily ignored.

"Why can't we move faster?" Nasrudin's employer asked him one day. "Every time I ask you to do something, you do it piecemeal. There is really no need to go to the market three times to buy three eggs."

Nasrudin promised to reform.

His master fell ill. "Call the doctor, Nasrudin."

The Mulla went out and returned, together with a horde of people. "Here, master, is the doctor. And I have brought the others as well."

"Who are all these others?"

"If the doctor should order a poultice, I have brought the poultice-maker, his assistant and the men who supply the ingredients, in case we need many poultices. The coalman is here to see how much coal we might need to heat water to make poultices. Then there is the undertaker, in case you do not survive."[1]

This tale is a caricature of our everyday experience. It serves to remind us that no one, at any time, can avoid the fact of death, and that most of us, at some time, will experience the process of dying.

Death and sex reflect a similar career. Each is crucial to one's sense of self. Each has been shrouded by a conspiracy of silence. Each is swamped with feelings of uncomfortableness. Each has seen its repulsive, obscene, and undesirable aspects driven into the open arena of unavoidable recognition.

The 1960s exploded with death: John F. Kennedy, Medgar Evers, Martin Luther King, Jr., Malcolm X, Robert Kennedy. These traumatized personal death. The Vietnam War intensified deper-sonalized death: body counts, atrocities, saturation bombing. The 1970s have aggravated the horror of death with mass murders, political terrorists, Attica uprisings. Yet one still stumbles over the experience of private death, as on the day I walked through Arlington National Cemetery with its row upon row upon row of white tablets. I was accompanying an army widow to Section 20, Plot 17, and the stone signaling her husband's grave. No matter where it comes or how it comes, death is everyone's burden!

It would not be inappropriate to mark 1965 as a turning point in our current grappling with death. Four theological students ap-proached Elisabeth Kübler-Ross requesting her aid in a project on dying as the biggest crisis people have to face. She suggested the tactic of asking dying patients: "What is it like? How does it feel? What fears, needs, fantasies do you have? What kind of things are we doing that are helpful? What kinds of things do we do that are detrimental?"

From that "happening" came her classic work on what the dying have to teach us. Subsequently, the ripeness of the times has seen consideration of dying and death made accessible and available to the public in general and to each of us individually.[2]

I will explore some of these commonly shared understandings of death and dying and then suggest directions for dealing with the event and the experience.

Understandings

The fact of death and the experience of dying are not single-face phenomena. They are many-sided realities.

Different Kinds

All dying is not the same.

Dying can be sudden and unexpected. A plane crashes. A car goes out of control. A sniper's bullet finds its mark. One moment a person is alive; the next moment the person is dead. A split second covers the transition from being alive to being dead.

Death can be anxiously anticipated and desperately fought. A soldier is ordered into battle. A patient is informed of the presence of a malignant and untreatable cancer. An intensely constricted span of time bridges the transition from being alive to being dead.

Or, death can be slow and drawn out. A patient with a degenerative disease attends to every little sign of the progressive loss of life. Old age eats away at the vital forces until one remains but a pale and fragile caricature of what one had been. A spaced-out wasteland connects the fertileness of being alive with the aridness of being dead. Death finally arrives as a relief from the relentless erosion of that which matters.

Just as all dying is not the same, so all death is not the same. Differences among the former are reciprocal to contrasts among the latter. When dying is sudden, death is tragic. When dying is excruciating, death is relief. When dying is quiet, death is consummation.

Death of the very young in no way corresponds to death of the very old. Death delayed may mean "partial" death or "bonus life." Death desired may mean bitter self-destruction or accepted self-completion. There are even a few who have died—technically—and returned to live another period.

Empirical investigation has related the variables of achievement, sex, age, and church attendance with nine theoretical perspectives on "The Meaning of Death."[3] The resulting factors were not given labels and I am supplying my own.

Factor 1—Death as Tragic: This was the first and strongest factor. It included very heavy emphasis on the perspectives of failure, loneliness, punishment, and pain in that order. It also included heavy emphasis on the perspective of forsaking dependents and some emphasis on death as unknown. The combinations of individual failure, interpersonal loss, and painful demise add up to the experience of dying and the fact of death as being "tragic."

Factor 2—Death with Confidence: This was the second strongest factor. It included very heavy emphasis on frequency of church attendance and the perspective of an afterlife of reward. It also included some emphasis upon the perspective of death as unknown, with a slight indication of women holding this combination more than men. The combination of institutional religious involvement and individual religious expectation suggests a confidence in the present that is anchored in eternity.

Factor 3—Death as Inevitable: The third factor produced a very heavy and virtually exclusive emphasis upon the variable of age. There was a slight negative correlation with the perspective of forsaking dependents. The older the person, the less death was likely to be seen as abandoning children. Death comes to all eventually.

Factor 4—Death with Courage: The final factor showed a fairly strong emphasis upon the perspective of death with courage and the variable of achievement. The perspective of death as a natural end also appeared with some emphasis in this factor. The courageous quality may be secular, humanistic, or religious, I am inclined to believe, but represents a focus on meeting the experience and the fact in contrast to the more confident focus on the beyond.

This analysis reveals the complexity of death as a symbol. It has multifaceted meanings. Death sharpens the tension between "there is still time" and "there is no more time," that is, the cutting off of possibilities, lost opportunities, unfulfilled experiences, the loss of power to participate in one's own destiny. It discloses the personal and subjective element behind the objective reality and event.

Death is inevitable.

Death can be tragic.

Death can be met with confidence anchored in a serene beyond and a certain present.

Death can be met with courage anchored in a substantial past and
an heroic present.

Additional analysis enables us to see even clearer the range of
individual reactions to the experience of dying and the fact of death.

Reactions

Despite the current notoriety of the topic, people still anxiously
avoid facing death.

Medical personnel, more than any other group, have constant and
sustained relationships with those who are traveling through the
valley of death. Unlike most of the population, they can avoid neither
the experience nor the fact. The very nature of their work puts them in
physical proximity to dying and death day in and day out. Their
reactions are but the reactions of the rest of us writ large.

Lawrence LeShan investigated the reaction of nurses whose
assignments kept them closest to death. With a stop watch, he timed
the interval between the moment a light appeared over the door of a
terminally ill patient and the moment a nurse entered the patient's
room in response. The results showed that the nurses tended to hurry
in response to lights of those who were less near death and that they
tended to drag their feet in response to lights of those who were more
near death. When LeShan inquired about the discrepancy, they
vigorously denied there was any. In their minds they were responding
to all patients in the same manner. They were completely unaware of
their avoidance and hesitancy. Evidently, he concluded, the discrepancy represents "an unconscious expression of their aversion to
death which had interfered with their care of their patients."[4]

The issue of informing patients about diagnosis and prognosis in
supposedly "hopeless" situations discloses a similar reaction of
anxious avoidance. In one survey of 444 physicians, it was found that
only 30 percent of them always or usually informed the patient, while
70 percent either never did or usually did not. Another survey found
that 90 percent preferred *not* telling the patient. A review of many
studies of research with doctors and patients showed that 69 to 90
percent of physicians favored *not* telling the patient of the possibility
of death. At the same time and in sharp contrast, 77 to 89 percent of
the patients wanted to know.[5]

The conclusion of one medical interpreter is strong:

In brief, we seem to be faced with the startling paradox that, as patients more and
more indicate a preference for being informed of the hopelessness of their situation,
physicians are becoming more and more reluctant to do so.[6]

Surely, one cannot be helpful to another if the other's pain keeps one's own nerves rubbed raw. It may be difficult to avoid developing "a practical callousness" as a means of staying close to death and dying without feeling overwhelmed. Some kind of distance is necessary, yet we need to distinguish between an accurate empathy that finds in the other what is in truth the other's experience and a sensitive sympathy that finds in the other what is in truth one's own experience. While everyone's death diminishes me, as the poet reminds us, and while each one's finitude is a reminder of my own finitude, another's death is not my death. And to make it so is to limit my helpful response to that human pain.

The anxious avoidance of death and dying by medical personnel only serves as an indicator of the reaction of most all of us. When we try to avoid the uncomfortableness, we still tend to be overwhelmed by the uncertainty. What can we say? How can we react? We find ourselves surrounding the dying person with a curtain of silence.

A fifty-one-year-old man suffering from severe coronary thrombosis had the following dream. In it he saw people gathered around a big hole in the middle of a green meadow. Everyone stood silently. The dreamer found the silence oppressive. He wondered why no one was talking. He was bothered by the fact that people were not shaking hands or interacting. Finally, he left in anger, determined never to see them or that place again.[7]

A forty-seven-year-old woman made that point more explicitly three weeks before she died of breast cancer. Everyone, she exclaimed, has "given me up. They have divorced themselves from me. They are even afraid to talk to me. If at least I could say goodbye to them."[8]

Each of these incidents is representative of our awkwardness in the presence of human death. Part of what presses us to shut out the other person's experience arises from our own guilt. We are relatively healthy and alive while the other is sick and dying. The contrast hurts everyone!

The silences that accompany anxiousness and uncertainty serve to isolate and alienate the living from the dying and the dying from the living. A touching response is destroyed. A distant (inhuman?) response metastasizes.

From having looked at those who only stand and wait, I want to compare the reactions of those who must meet and master the reality sooner rather than later. What is the experience like for the one who is dying? What does he or she go through? Here is where the work of Kübler-Ross assists us.

From interviews with hundreds of terminally ill patients, Kübler-Ross has constructed a map of the territory individuals cover in their final journey. Five stages are identifiable:

1. denial and isolation, in which an individual buffers the anticipated end with a "not me" attitude;
2. anger, in which an individual rages against the anticipated end with a "why me" attitude;
3. bargaining, in which an individual attempts to postpone the anticipated end by a magical "if it doesn't come now, then I will do such-and-such" attitude;
4. depression, in which an individual responds to the anticipated end with feelings of great loss in a "what's the use" attitude;
5. acceptance, in which an individual comes to acknowledge the anticipated end as one's own with a "yes, me" attitude.[9]

These stages may come close together or be spaced somewhat apart. It is not clear whether everyone goes through each stage or may skip one or more of them. What is clear, however, is the desirable transition from a destructive avoidance to a constructive acceptance.

It is for that transition that most of us need suggestions. How can one respond touchingly rather than distantly? What is helpful and what is harmful? How can the experience of dying and the fact of death become expressions of genuine identity and real integrity?

How, in short, ought we to deal with the last human limit and the inevitable human end?

Directions

Death and dying force upon us a certain honesty about life and living. Where truth is lacking in living, truth will be lacking in dying. In fact, life and death appear related: the more life the easier death; the less life the more terrible death. I do not mean these in the physical and literal sense, but rather in the human and figurative sense. In the face of finitude we find ourselves driven to deal with our work, our worth, our love, our life.

What is most terrifying about dying and death is the lack of a living connectedness. Without presence, we are without hope; without contact, we are without grounding. So we find we are required to face what separates the living from the dying. We find we are required to face our own limits and our own end. For we, too, will die. In facing death we are finding life. And in finding life we establish a living connectedness. We come closer to one another for mutual gratification and upbuilding.

The Demand to "Be"

Perhaps no other experience accentuates this demand as much as the inadequacy of "doing" and the necessity for "being." To be able to "do" something tends to reduce uncomfortableness and to hold out hope of change. To have to "be" someone tends to heighten uncomfortableness and to imply no change. This means to let be, to allow to be, to accept what is as it is. To do means to interfere, to alter, to go beyond what is to what might be. In the presence of the last dividing line, the only thing we can do is to be.

The courage to be is inseparably linked with the courage to be known.[10] The existential demand upon each of us individually has its accompanying interpersonal demand. I can be courageous if I can communicate to a significant other what matters desperately to me. Communication constitutes the core of the doing of being. When I can say to you what I am experiencing, then we have entered into a transforming communion. Distance disappears. Loneliness lessens. Isolation is swallowed up by oneness. As I am known, so I am I.

Now is the time. Here is the place. What one person says to another in the face of death counts more intensely than in any other here-and-now. The one who is anticipating the end wants to be heard, aches to be understood, longs to be in touch. There is a heightened awareness that every word matters, each moment counts, every gesture carries special weight. The quality of the connectedness replaces the quantity of the connections. A sense of eternity comes with experiencing being known by another and knowing the other right here/right now.

Over the last seven years of my father's life, there were several occasions when death loomed imminently. Each time we talked some about our lives and our relationship. On one occasion I wrote him a letter (since he was in Phoenix, Arizona, and I in Rochester, New York). Months later he answered me. My letter had meant "so very much" to him and there were some things he wanted to say, "though I think you know without my saying anything."

Even when we "know without having to say," it is important to have said it explicitly at least some of the time. I share a somewhat extended section of his letter for several reasons. First, the letter expresses the struggle and pain that so often accompany dying.

Second, it affirms the desire to matter that is a part of so many. Third, it illustrates my point about the demand to be rather than to do in such moments.

> You gave me credit for so much courage and said you would think I would wish it were all over and I didn't have to suffer anymore. Countless times I have felt that. I have very little courage of my own. I know that such an attitude is wrong and one certainly cannot pray about it. As a matter of fact, one cannot know when he should live and when he should go. He can, however, pray for strength and courage and grace to meet whatever proves to be the experience. That I have done, or I don't see how I could have gotten through these past few years.
>
> I think the worst of all was the first few days of this last time in the hospital. They seemed unendurable. When one thinks of words to describe them, the words "kaleidoscopic hell" are the only ones that come to mind. Without prayer I don't see how I could have endured them.

Then he goes on to speak more specifically of the "being" element in our relationship.

> The thing that meant so very much to me, Jim, was your understanding of me enough to know that you could say what you did then—that it looked as though we were heading for a crisis, you hoped and prayed it might be for the better, but you realized it might be for the worse.
>
> You are the only person who seems to know me well enough to know that you could say that. The fact that we have been able to show our love and affection for each other is one of the precious things of life. You referred to our having faced the ultimate issues of life together. I felt, too, that we have and yet you know very little was put into words.

From the more personal and intimate issue of our relationship, Dad went on to express something of his experience of facing the fact of death. Again, what he shares is not unique to him but quite common, as Kübler-Ross's fifth stage of acceptance suggests.

> One thing I have found is that once you have faced what was almost certain death, there is a release and a peace one never experienced before. Whether one is to live or die at any other time is almost immaterial. Whatever comes is all right and one really has no concern.

Doing ceases. Only being remains.

The Demand to Humanize

The "being" character of the experience clearly emphasizes the *human* response of the participants. Instead of becoming less personal, we are required to become more personal. What we could gloss over in other circumstances can no longer be avoided. Whereas we may have seen each other through a glass darkly, now we are to attend to each other "face to face." The transition from a negative to a positive event requires our human presence.

Of what does human presence consist?

The end *and* the means of human presence are truth in the situation. There is to be as much full human contact as possible. What we say and what we do is communication in search of communion. We intentionally seek a relationship. There is no dignity and no courage in deception. The "isness" of dying calls out in all its fullness. If we have known only a fraction of the truth previously, now we are to know it as fully as is humanly possible. For that is the heart of love, and, as Paul reminds us, faith and hope somehow have their grounding in love (see 1 Corinthians 13:13). The issue is not whether we share what is happening. Instead the issue is *how* we share what is happening.

Truth that looms so awesome in anticipation looks so simple in retrospect. What we felt would damage and destroy, we discover actually helps and heals. We saw that with Rhonda's parts and pieces. We see it also in the experience of dying. But *how* to see that reality and *how* to get to that truth seem so complicated.

Again Kübler-Ross has shown us a way. One does not want unfeelingly to bombard the dying person with "the" fact: "You're dying." Nor does one want unfeelingly to avoid the fact by asserting: "You're going to be all right." Rather one wants to find a way to say what is. And she provides an opening.

"How sick are you?"

A simple question; a "door opening" response; the opportunity for genuine give-and-take.[11] It does not force presence where one prefers privacy. It does not perpetuate privacy where one wants presence. It does not "do" where doing is uncalled for. Instead it allows. It helps to be. It lets life flow. It creates a genuinely human relationship.

With such an invitation from the living, the dying can say "what is" for them. That may be much; it may be little. It matters less. What does matter is the reaching out in love. We help the dying by responding to their life situation as *theirs*. They may still be in a state of shocked denial. They may have moved into bitterness and envy. They may engage in magical maneuverings, negotiating now for this and now for that. They may be staggered by the loss of livelihood and life and love. They may have found the peace that nothing can dislodge. What is important is not what they are experiencing but rather that we be present to them in their experience.

As we talk, we share.

As we share, we care.

As we care, we give courage.

Most people dread the process of dying more than the fact of death. Death for the elderly usually comes with a sense of appropriate completion of the life lived. In stark contrast, dying for the elderly looms as a sheer catastrophe. One anticipates—and not without considerable evidence of its occurrence—dying without dignity. There comes a time when one no longer has control over one's self, one's bodily functioning, one's interpersonal world. There comes a time when one dreads being taken over by an impersonalized and dehumanizing environment.

Clinging obsessively to life conveys for me a fundamental denial of the meaningfulness of living. The character of the life being lived always takes precedence over the mere fact of life itself. There is no dignity in prolonging a vegetable existence. There is nothing redemptive in unmitigated suffering. Endless existing as a value means empty living as a consequence.

The demand to humanize dying finds its most acute implication in maintaining for the one dying a sense of continuation with his or her experience of healthy life. Here one is treated as a living person, one who is respected, cared for, shared with, turned to, relied upon. In place of the curtain of silence, there is a sphere of sharing. If one errs in taking the dying person's own wishes and feelings into account in making decisions and carrying on activities, one errs on the side of "more likely" to take these into account rather than less likely to take these into account. The dying person is encouraged to possess as much real psychic space as possible. Even if the choice is limited to wearing "this" hair ribbon or "that" hair ribbon, the right to be part of the process is protected. Concrete decisions and specific acts are what enable people to continue to experience themselves as a part of life. Through such experiences people feel that they are sharing in the continuing flow of life.

A sense of continuity requires an anticipated confidence that what one has known before the transition one will surely know through the transition. A twenty-eight-year-old white Catholic mother, hospitalized with a terminal liver disease, put the need well. Kübler-Ross had been sitting with her. As the woman held her hand, she said, "You have such warm hands. I hope you are going to be with me when I get colder and colder." [12]

In *human* presence there is hope, even for those who are dying right here / right now.

The Demand for Meaning

Unlike other animals, we humans are not simply shaped by events. We shape events. We alone know the split between "what's there" and the meaning that "isness" has for us. Of all creatures we alone must determine the significance of whatever happens.

What is true in living is equally true in dying. What does my death mean to me? How does my death influence me? What will my death be like?

In *The Book of Common Prayer* there is a prayer in the midst of which is this phrase: "Deliver us from sudden death." Similarly, the psalmist (39:4) calls out to God: "let me know my end." The point of these petitions is a plea that death not come prematurely and without warning.[13] We want some time to assimilate the reality of certain death. We want enough time to act wisely in relation to the responsibilities that are ours. We want time to learn to die. We want to participate in and own that which is at hand.

In the summer of 1972, my family and I were in Japan. An urgent letter arrived from my mother. She was to have had a routine cataract operation, but it had been unexpectedly canceled. She wanted me to get in touch with her as soon as possible. I telephoned her from Hawaii. Her physician had discovered she was suffering from multiple myeloma, a cancer of the bone marrow. Because of this he had canceled the operation. Even more, this meant she had about five months to live. Instead of returning home, I immediately went to see her.

Like so many courageous souls whose petition to be delivered from sudden death is answered, mother prepared herself. She had been cleaning out closets, going through boxes, straightening up records somewhat persistently prior to her fatal illness. She had known that she would die someday, but that day had seemed far off. So she had been proceeding with the certain yet muffled truth of finitude. Now she faced the certain and stark truth of her impending death. Overnight, the cleaning out, going through, straightening up took on an urgency. If she did not do it now, it would not be done.

After her death, we found a postcard she had sent to a friend two weeks after she learned of her disease and four months before it consumed her. She had written a single sentence. It stated what was. It sounded her courage. It read: "I told you there might not be much time left; well, there isn't!"

There was not much time, but enough to enable her to know her end. She made plans, with care and with thoroughness. She settled her affairs. She engaged in activities that mattered to her—being with friends, seeing all the family, working on the election, speaking on behalf of the United Nations, arranging contacts between people significant to her and the causes to which she gave herself, having an informal gathering in which I could share some of my impressions of Japan. She did what she wanted, as much as she could, for as long as she could. She continued to cross lines and lives, linking diversity into a mosaic of splendid humanity.

The day came when she no longer could do what she wanted. She moved from her apartment to the infirmary at her retirement home and then to the hospital. Her time was up. She knew the ravages the disease would inflict on her and the heartache her excruciating pain would cause for those who loved her. Deliberately, she chose to stop eating. Nourishment would only prolong the inevitable. She took just enough liquid to prevent any added complications caused by dehydration. She had settled her affairs. She had lived her life. She had been graced with time to know her end.

In our last conversation, she spoke of what lay ahead in light of what had gone before. "In the next world I will try to take more time to read." A rather frivolous remark on the threshold of eternity, yet it reflected her own restless involvement in being and doing with others for the sake of life and love. She also planned to take time "to explore the planets." Her curiosity continued to the end.

Then she spoke her final blessing. "I give you Charlie's sense of humor." Charlie is an uncle on my father's side who has always been the jovial member of the family. In her own quiet, unassuming, and heroically humorous way she was saying: "I give you my sense of humor, my ability to see life in ways others do not, my genius at putting others at ease, and my gift of lifting a bit the burdens others bear." She would never have been so bold as to have thought, much less have said, such things about herself. But to me that is what she meant: "I bestow upon you my gift to transcend!"

She gave me—and others—far more than I knew earlier and fortunately realized while she was still alive: love, vision, care, concern for peace and purpose, craziness, imagination, laughter, warmth, relationships—life itself!

And so she died.

It is easy to acknowledge intellectually the fact of death. It is more difficult to know experientially the closeness of dying. Sometimes we are given tastes of such timing. A close call. A critical diagnosis. A serious operation. For a brief period the intensity of eternity replaces the ongoingness of time. Life stands out—sharply, sensitively, compellingly. We know our end. We can shape the meaning of what is happening.

In the early years of my ministry, I would find myself torn apart by contrasting experiences of a wedding and a funeral on the same day. Somehow the inevitable intrusion of death muffled the delightful celebration of life. I no longer feel torn. Oh, I can experience the joyfulness of a wedding and I can experience the painfulness of a funeral, but I no longer see them as contradictory.

A tearful accepting in these later years has replaced the desperate resisting of my early years. Whether one is young or old, whether one has lived much or lived little, whether death is completion or disruption, I have come upon a deeper quality. And that quality is this: there has been someone rather than no one; there has been something rather than nothing. And the pain of having lost does not need to diminish the joy of having had. Death is lifted up and thereby becomes part of our truly human destiny.

Death is a fact of life. It is natural, unavoidable, inevitable. Within the scheme of creation we alone know that we are going to die. That is our freedom; this is our finitude. Our faith always looks beyond our own little lives to the larger life in God. We are creatures—limited, finite, mortal. In the book of Genesis the recital of the lives of the patriarchs always ends with the same refrain: "Thus all the days of _____ were [so many] years; and he died." Nowhere are we promised reprieve.

Belief in immortality of the soul inappropriately suggests that there is something within us that does not die.

More accurately, the doctrine of the resurrection of the body expresses both our human limitations and God's potentialities. It acknowledges that death is death—crucified, dead, and buried, as the Apostles' Creed puts it. It recognizes that we are not isolated atoms, but part of the whole fabric of the universe—all are restored to meaningful relatedness. It insists that we are not split between a good immortal soul and a bad prisonhouse body—the whole person dies, the whole person triumphs. Even more, it affirms that in life there is always more than my own or anyone else's presence. Our best is never good enough to avoid unintended negative consequences. Our worse is never bad enough to prevent something being salvageable by God. With forgiveness those realities worth preserving are sustained within the economy of that which neither moth nor rust can consume.

That which matters most does not ultimately go down the drain. Life and love are not "nectar in a sieve."

The intensity that floods us in the presence of death and dying ought to remind us of the essence of life and living.

Even dying, which is most individual, takes place in the context of community. The painful loneliness of unconnected living mirrors the painful loneliness of unconnected dying. Only human responding can heal that most human hurt.

Thus, Dr. Charles Mayo of the famed Mayo Clinic voiced what I suspect is the deep hope of every one of us: "When I die, I hope someone I love will hold my hand."

In death—as in life—sorrow is great; closeness is greater; love is greatest!

A LARGER TASK

Garcin: . . . now suppose we start trying to help each other.

Inez: I don't need help.

Garcin: Inez, they've laid their snare damned cunningly—like a cobweb. If you make any movement, if you raise your hand to fan yourself, Estelle and I feel a little tug. Alone, none of us can save himself or herself; we're linked together inextricably. So you can take your choice.

Jean Paul Sartre, *No Exit* [1]

10

The Use of Others:
resources and referrals

Thus far I have dealt with deep issues of meaning—parts and pieces, dependency, aging, dying—and primarily with an individual therapeutic approach to helping—grammar and guts, beginning with ourselves. In the remainder of the book I will shift the focus of the approach to human pain. Whereas I have emphasized the helper and the "helpee" in immediate and intimate interaction, I want now to enlarge the company of helpers and then to redefine what effective response can mean.

This chapter will be a nuts-and-bolts discussion of how we can use others to help us in responding to pain. In the next chapter I will look at the structures and systems in which individuals are embedded as the central focus of responding.

Why Don't We Use Others?

Generally, clergypersons have not used helping resources in their communities. In the report of the Joint Commission on Mental Health,[2] it was disclosed that people seeking help about emotional or psychological problems appealed to the clergy more frequently than any other resource. Forty-two percent reported turning first to the clergy, and sixty-four percent of these were satisfied with the help they received.[3] It appeared they preferred the clergy because there was less demand for introspection. They looked for emotional support rather than personality change. Their interpersonal difficulties could be seen in less psychological terms. There was less implicit demand for change in themselves.

In reviewing the pattern, the Commission went on to point out: "The helping process seems to stop with the [clergypersons]." Even though more than one-third of the counseling problems dealt with by clergy were estimated to have serious psychiatric dimensions, only one in ten persons was referred.[4]

Clergy appear to function very much on their own. They draw on support from neither helping resources in the community nor their own colleagues.[5] The emerging picture, however, is not one of clergy "with serene confidence in religion, in the church, in themselves when confronted with mental health problems, but rather of [professionals] in a dilemma: considerable ambivalence about the efficacy of religious resources, and at the same time reservations and anxiety about referring parishioners to psychiatrists and other professional resources. Serious barriers to communication, to understanding, to perception seem to exist between [clergyperson] and psychiatrist, between [clergyperson] and parishioner, and often between [clergyperson] and [clergyperson]."[6] Clergy feel alienated and alone among helping professionals.

While clergy seldom use community resources, the need for their using them is great. Clergy stand in the center of community life and are free to take initiative with people in pain. They can go anywhere, be anywhere, move around anywhere without having to explain or justify their presence. Few professionals are privileged with as much freedom of movement. In time of stress people first turn to the clergy more than other professionals. The need for professional support and the desirability of special skills ought to encourage clergy to work collaboratively with other helping persons.

Yet, consider barriers that appear to be inherent in the clergy's inability to take advantage of community services. Not only may one fear that one's pastoral role might be lost, but one seems to fear that the role of religion in the life of the person suffering might be lost. The minister may view other helping professions as antagonistic or indifferent to religion. Thus, by referring a parishioner outside the religious setting, the minister "gives up" a responsibility that he or she deeply cherishes.

The minister also fears that the parishioner may not find a sympathetic and personal response at the referral service. One caseworker reported:

> Our bad reputations seem linked in part with our harried tempo, our not always taking the time to hear clients out to the point where we can make an adequate disposition of the case. Despite our concentration on making careful referrals, clients still complain of having sought service in an Agency and of having been seen by a worker for only ten minutes before being directed to another Agency, which was still unable to meet the request. Clients are sensitive about being rejected and are inclined to magnify even one negative experience when they are in a position of enforced dependency. Asking for help brings hostile feelings close to the surface.[7]

Furthermore, the clergyperson may feel there is a stigma attached to a person using community services. There may be connotations of sickness, pathology, charity, handout, failure. To the degree I have feelings of apprehension and ambivalence about community services, the parishioner will feel a sense of stigma.

The clergy's sense of guilt may act as another barrier to using community resources. Though one experiences being over one's head and wants very much to get rid of the individual, a basic desire to help may cause one to hang on to the relationship with the vague hope that problems will eventually resolve themselves. The clergyperson may not want to admit that more help is needed by the individual than he or she can give.

What Resources Are Available?

Consider now "what" we mean by community resources. There are two kinds, neither is exclusive, yet each has its own emphasis. They are the psychological and the sociological.

Psychological services deal primarily with the self in its own right. The focus is on psychological dynamics, the structure and function of the personality.

Sociological services focus primarily on the self in its social context. The emphasis is upon social dynamics, the person in his or her situation and in his or her interpersonal interactions.

I shall deal with these two later in considering when to refer. At present they simply provide two convenient vantage points from which to view community services. It is understood, however, that all community services combine both psychological and sociological dimensions in their work.

Basic community services may be grouped under five general categories:

1. *Financial assistance to meet basic needs:* old age assistance, aid to dependent children who lack support, care, or guidance of one or both parents; aid to the disabled, who experience permanent impairment preventing earning of an income or running a household; aid to the blind; general assistance to those whose needs are not covered elsewhere; Social Security, including old-age and survivor's insurance; and unemployment compensation.

2. *Family and child welfare services:* family agencies; Traveler's Aid, which helps transients looking for greater opportunity by assisting with more realistic plans; child welfare services, including protective services and services where families are temporarily or permanently broken up; adoption services; services for unwed mothers; institutional care for retarded or disturbed children; and day care.

3. *Educational and recreational services:* Y programs, scouts, and social work groups.

4. *Health services:* hospitals and clinics, including both physical and psychological services.

5. *Services for the aging.*[8]

The scope of community services is staggering. The National Conference on Social Welfare has approximately twelve hundred agencies and sixty associate groups connected with it. While the pattern of community services including both public and private services varies from area to area, one may assume there is some kind of local council coordinating the services.

Such an overview is crucial. Information as to the number, variety, and accessibility is basic.

Beyond information as to what services are available, the helper needs to develop a network of professional and personal contacts. The contacts are to be not only with agencies but also with personnel. Similarly, there needs to be contact with those individuals who provide psychological and sociological resources privately.

Services ought to be evaluated before they are used. One needs to ask: who sponsors the agency or the person, what is the training required for the helping person, what is the reputation of the service, does one feel one has enough information about the service that one can direct a person to it with a fair degree of confidence?

When to Use Others

When the clergyperson confronts someone in need, he or she has to assess what the need is before action can be taken. One begins by constructing a working image of the person with whom one is talking. "He seems to be the sort of person who. . . ." One focuses on the facts of the situation. "The facts appear to be. . . ." One explores possible alternatives to meet the need. One evolves a plan that the sufferer hopefully will see as being concerned with his or her welfare. Let me illustrate what I mean by assessment before action.

A thirty-one-year-old married woman comes to me as a result of increasing stress in her home and increasing inability to function. She has been married thirteen years; there are five children. Her husband was hospitalized for an acute depression a year and a half after they were married. Subsequently, he had a number of recurrences of the depressive pattern. Until the preceding few months, she had played the dominant role in the family. She made the decisions and carried the responsibility. She did that, she indicates, because of her feeling that he was unable to. Within the past year she has established her first close friendships with two women through a small group in the church. As a result, she has begun to feel she has someone who cares about her. She carries on long telephone conversations with these two women.

Six months previously she introduced her husband to Recovery, Inc. That is a group similar to AA but made up of former mental hospital patients. Within three weeks he began to change. Whereas he had been weak, now he became stronger; whereas he had allowed her to carry the masculine role, now he began assuming the masculine role. He was concerned with handling the money and disciplining the children. He even went so far as to restrict her to home. Now she is feeling vulnerable, less able to deal with life. Not only are roles reversed, but she feels undermined in her adequacy as a person.

I would be uncomfortable in dealing with this situation on my own. The persisting depressive pattern of the husband has a dangerous quality. The dramatic reversal of marital roles suggests serious personality disturbances. The financial needs of the family appear to be complicated. The combination would be more than I would care to handle. Therefore, I would quickly consider how to use other resources in the community.

Three pieces emerge as salient in assessing possible referral. First, there is the depressive pattern of the husband. That suggests the helping person ought to have psychiatric know-how and access to psychiatric facilities. Second, there is the marital conflict and the role conflict. That suggests someone specializing in the intricacies of marital relationships. Third, there is the woman's dependency and loneliness as revealed in her relationship with women. That suggests the desirability of a woman. In putting these three pieces together, I concluded that a certain woman psychiatric social worker, in part-time private practice, might be the most appropriate referral. She is associated with the out-patient clinic of one of the psychiatric hospital facilities. She specializes in marital and family conflict. She can give active support to the woman, as well as mobilizing other resources in case of an emergency. As a result of a careful assessment, an appropriate use of others can be made.

Consider now the two foci of community services—psychological and sociological—in assessing the need for referral action.

Indicators of need for referral to psychological resources are both obvious and subtle. Most simply, I would say they are present whenever we find disturbances in the basic functioning of a person— in one's sleeping, in one's eating, in one's working, in one's communicating, in one's relating. Whenever the behavior of an individual changes unexpectedly and radically, whenever the behavior is bizarre and unusual, whenever the behavior is dangerous to the person and to others, whenever anxiety is disproportionate to reality factors, referral is indicated.

The necessity for sociological referrals grows out of more situational, relational, and concrete problems. In a sense, social welfare agency services fall to those "in-between" people "who are not clamoring to have help in becoming more adequate . . . but who are not neglectful enough to fall within the province of the protective agency."[9] In such situations there is need for professional services ranging from what may be relatively simple, concrete service to a more complex involvement in family attitudes and reluctance to secure help.

Consider services needed when a young woman comes indicating that she is pregnant and unmarried.[10] Marriage is not necessarily the only or even the desirable answer. If adoption is an alternative, the helper needs to be aware of the social welfare agencies involved in such work. Facilities for the unmarried pregnant young woman vary. There are maternity homes, foster homes, recommended boarding homes. All are within reach of adequate clinical facilities and have qualified social casework services available. There may also be need for legal counsel.

In addition to disturbances in a person's basic functioning or situational and concrete problems, four general matters ought also to be noted in deciding when and how to use others:

1. The work of a clergyperson embraces many functions. Pastoral care and pastoral counseling are only part of one's work. One cannot carry everyone; one cannot cover everyone. One's job requires a skillful balancing of many demands and much pain.

2. After seeing a person three or four times, if no progress is discernible, one should probably consult with other professional services. As a general rule, a minister ought not to spend more than ten or twelve hours a week in ministering to specific individuals on a counseling basis. Anyone requiring help over a long period of time needs to be referred to those whose jobs specifically focus on such pain.

3. Whenever a clergyperson begins to feel in deep water, out over one's head and floundering, one ought to begin the referral process. Such uncomfortableness indicates there are elements in the situation beyond one's competence and control. Clergy have a tendency to be too self-sufficient. There is more of a demand on their own inner resources than is true of most other professionals. It is precisely at moments of uncomfortableness that we ought to be participating in shared ministry.

4. While the skills of the clergy are varied and while each has unique skills, nevertheless, the clergyperson is a generalist in the midst of increasing specialization. Not only is it unrealistic, but also inappropriate, to expect him or her to be aware of and to be able to carry out the variety of services necessary to minister to people in the complex patterns of modern society. The utilization of other people in the helping process is not so much a sign of pastoral failure as a sign of pastoral wisdom. In many ways the clergyperson is the facilitator, the encourager, the director, the introducer,[11] the clarifier within the community. The role is to ask: What needs are foremost? Who can best help? How may that help be made available? The role is that of servant.

Having looked at why we tend not to use others and at what resources are available and at when we ought to use others, let's explore how we can use others in responding to human pain.

Bridging the Referral Gap

How can we take advantage of resources in the community? How does one go about the job? How may the person being referred see the process as something concerned with his or her welfare?[12]

The referral process requires, as I have implied, distinguishing between the person and the problem on the one hand and the service and the referral on the other. The process may be seen as building a bridge across a river. On one side stands the person who is to be referred and the reason he or she needs to be referred. On the other bank lies the community service—what it is and where it is. The question is, "How do we bridge that gap?" How do we link the person with the possibility?

The construction of the referral bridge may be thought of as a three-stage process: intervention, interpretation, and introduction.

Intervention

Consider first the matter of intervention. Clergy operate in a largely uncontrolled milieu. There are few external structures to bring people to one or to keep people with one. People come and go as they please. Yet unlike other professionals, clergy are free to take initiative. They may go to people wherever they are without having to explain or justify their presence. They may make themselves available by putting themselves in physical proximity to people. That physical proximity may turn into personal presence. The only power which clergy possess is the moral power of their person and the faith they represent.

Because of the ambiguity in clergy relationships, intervention is not easy. After one makes contact with a hurting person, one has to move beyond empathic support to more confrontational direction. Alan Keith-Lucas has suggested statements he has found helpful in responding to those in need.[13] They can be of assistance in the task of intervention. The statements are:

"*This is it.*" This is the real situation, stripped of all its polite coverings—what you are really up against.

"*I know that it hurts.*" As far as it is given to me, I feel for you and with you in facing this trouble; and anytime you want to bring out—your anger, your fear, or your doubts, it will be acceptable to me—not because I feel them myself, but because I know that I could feel them.

"*I will stand by you to help you if you want me.*" I will not force you, but at the same time nothing will shake my willingness to help you should you ask it of me.

Intervention, then, is offering another an opportunity to change oneself and/or one's situation by the use of something growing out of the relationship. It requires of the other admitting inadequacies, insufficiencies, and failures in one's life. It requires that one put oneself in the power of another person by letting the other know one's true situation. It requires not one decision, but an endless chain of decisions. It means risking a painful yet known past for an unknown and uncertain future. The suggestion has been made, not without validity, that this process of receiving help has dynamics rooted deeply in religious experience.[14] Repentance, submission, steadfastness under temptation, and faith are all present in such a helping relationship.

Interpretation

The intervention phase of building the referral bridge moves rapidly into the interpretation phase. As the situation has been clarified, possible directions and necessary decisions emerge.

To mobilize the person's motivation for referral is a delicate art. The other must be experiencing enough discomfort that he or she wants to begin doing something to change. One needs to be aware of alternatives. One needs confidence in one's own ability to pursue an appropriate alternative and to reach the objective of modifying that which is causing the discomfort. One needs to recognize that "change is apt to be a slow process; it is marked by hesitation to move from the known to the unknown, and a tendency to fall back upon familiar patterns of behavior."[15]

To the degree the sufferer sees the locus of responsibility and initiative lying within oneself and one's interaction with the situation, one will be able to mobilize oneself.

The key to helpful interpretation appears to be the ability to mobilize the inner resources of individuals to participate in their own destinies. Rather than the helper being the expert diagnostician and prescriber of solutions, the helper explores with them the nature of the situation, possible alternatives, and ways of pursuing an appropriate direction. At that point, we, the helpers, are not seeking dramatic changes in the others' lives. We are content if we are able to affect a slight change in the direction in which they are going.[16] After a while, a minimum shift in direction has a major effect in what happens, just as a directional modification of a boat on a lake makes a difference in where one lands.

To assist an individual in understanding the directions in which one might move, in making the decision for a particular direction, and in acting on it requires that the helper understand the obstacles involved. We assume—almost without qualification—that the other will have mixed feelings about getting help. Part of the person wants help and part does not. Part of the person looks forward to coming and part does not. There are no easy answers; there are no pat solutions; there is no great messiah who is going to make everything all right by magic or majesty. There is no quick or easy way to work through a person's ambivalence about receiving help. Feelings both of wanting help and of resisting help need to be respected.

To the helper looking on in another's life, the direction may be obvious. To the person struggling with his or her own situation, direction may be far from obvious. The security operations by which one maintains oneself in the face of the demands of the environment are not easily modified. Anxiety has a way of crippling an individual's ability to respond. The more fully the helper enables the sufferer to clarify conflicts within oneself, resistance to securing help, and hostility against the person trying to help, the easier will be the referral.

For example, a parishioner comes seeking information as to possible nursing home care for an aged parent. On the surface that may be simply an informational matter. What nursing homes are available, both private and public? What public health nursing assistance may be available to the aged in one's own home? What financial resources are available under the Public Assistance Division of the Department of Social Welfare?

Underlying these informational questions, however, are the attitudes and feelings of the person. The ability of the parishioner to use the community services as fully and as appropriately as possible depends upon his or her being helped to face the negatives in the situation. There probably is a genuine caring for the parent and a desire to help. At the same time the problems of the aging become so complex that resentment grows as one has to care for the one who is increasingly unable to care for herself or himself. There is resentment at being constricted by the increasingly narrowed existence of the parent. There is uncomfortableness or guilt over one's own feelings of annoyance. There is embarrassment in allowing another to see the negativism. There is sensitivity to the way neighbors, friends, and family are viewing the way the parent is being taken care of.

So the simple question of referral information takes place in a context of attitudes and feelings that require facing the negatives in order to free the person to pursue the possibilities.

A sense of timing is a crucial element in interpretation. An extended period of a supporting relationship may be necessary as preparation for actually utilizing community services. In some instances, particularly with the chronically emotionally disturbed, that period may stretch out for months. In other instances, the supporting relationship may be established in one contact. Clergypersons seem to err in opposite directions in the referral process. As I indicated above, they tend not to refer as often as they ought. At the same time, they tend to be overly eager to refer in certain situations.

An overeagerness to refer may reflect lack of faith in one's own competence. It may reveal one's desire to avoid a messy relationship. One is only too ready to pass on a headache.

In interpreting the individual's need for referral, the clergyperson has to clarify his or her own limitations in the relationship. Rather than saying, "I have taken you as far as I can go now" or "You are too hot to handle," he or she may suggest, "Let's see what other possibilities there might be for help on this problem." [17] In acknowledging one's limitations, the helper endeavors to assist the individual to see the situation that way. As the individual understands the boundaries, he or she is more able to explore other sources of assistance.

Referral does not mean desertion, yet it may be perceived that way. After a clergyperson had made a referral to a family service agency, for instance, the person became uneasy. Exploration of the feelings revealed the fear that the clergyperson was deserting him. By that he meant that he and his wife would simply be passed on from one agency to another without anyone ever helping them face their difficulty. He wanted assurance from the clergyperson that there would be an ongoing support throughout the process.

Part of ongoing support involves interpreting the individual's relationship with the referral service. It is not unusual for the sufferer to return to the clergyperson with distressing stories of negligence, indifference, and mishandling on the part of the agency to which he or she was referred. It is hazardous to take such reports at face value. People resent dependent relationships. Consequently, they easily respond in distorted and illogical ways. Rather than rising up in righteous indignation at the impersonal bureaucracy or individual incompetency of the referral service, the clergyperson needs to interpret the intricacies of the helping relationship. He or she can accept the individual's feelings of anger, hurt, and resentment. He or she can encourage the individual to be more aware of ambivalences and reluctance to be helped.

The clergyperson needs definitely to encourage the individual to return to the referral service and talk through the difficulty in that relationship. One may say something like this: "I regret that you are finding the process so upsetting. I appreciate your feeling that you can share with me what seems to be happening. I wonder if, as a result of our talking together, you can go back and tell the worker exactly how you are feeling. Could you tell him you feel he isn't really listening to you? Could you let him know you feel he is trying to push you around? I know he would appreciate having the honest feedback, for unless you let him know what you are experiencing, he will not be able to assist you as you need." We can encourage the distressed person to go back and deal with the distress directly.

So far, in constructing the referral bridge, I have dealt with the initial phase of intervention in an individual's life situation and the second phase of interpretation, both interpretation of the need for referral and interpretation that is a part of the ongoing supporting relationship. I turn now to the third phase, namely, the introduction of the person to the referral service.

Introduction

To introduce people to each other, we need to know the people we are introducing. The more we know about people, the easier it is to introduce them. The clergyperson ought not to wait until an emergency to become acquainted with services in the community. Not only does one need an overall knowledge of the health, welfare, and recreation services, one also needs personal knowledge. Any referral process is facilitated if it takes place within an already established network of professional and personal contacts.

Such contacts may be developed in various ways. The helper may visit a particular service with the express purpose of becoming acquainted with its staff, its setting, and its functioning. As one takes part in various community organizations, one has opportunity to meet other helping persons. One might invite such individuals to lunch for the purpose of becoming acquainted and sharing professional concerns. Most professionals with whom I am acquainted are receptive to and desirous of such working relationships.

Out of accumulated contacts, the clergyperson begins to develop personal knowledge not only of helping services but of helping persons. Thus in making a referral one may indicate, "I know so-and-so who works at that agency. We have had contact and I have a good deal of confidence in him."

The more the helper knows a particular service or helping person, the more appropriate will be the referral. Thus one will understand the strengths and limitations of each service. One will not give the impression that any specialist or agency has all the answers. Most people mistakenly conceive the referral process as a mechanical operation in which some impersonal need is matched by some impersonal answer. Referral ought to be understood as a process similar to firing a high-powered rifle rather than simply firing a shotgun. Each agency or specialist tends to have certain kinds of strengths as well as certain weaknesses. Experience gives the helper information as to the potential of each service to help.

A clarification of expectations is essential. What may the person expect and not expect? It is our responsibility to avoid preparing people for services which simply do not exist. As one caseworker commented, "Many of us have experienced, on both the giving and receiving end, the type of wishful thinking which imbues others with superhuman powers to give help when we are unable to go further or when the situation is inoperable." [18] There are no magic helpers; there are no pat answers; there is no easy solution. Referral has to be grounded in reality.

The helper, therefore, introduces the individual to as many of the concrete procedures as possible. Intake will include the following: (1) focusing on and clarifying the problems for which the individual is seeking help; (2) evaluating what the individual has already tried to do in meeting the situation; (3) assessing the motivation of the individual for utilizing the help of the service and identifying resistances and reservations; (4) deciding whether or not the service one wants is available under the conditions which one can accept.[19] There is the matter of cost. Is it free or is there some kind of a sliding scale, and if so, what are the minimum and maximum levels expected? Most services are overworked. Consequently, there may be a waiting list of those who have been declared eligible but who must wait until personnel are available. In short, a clarification of the limits in the referral resource enables the individual to be clearer as to the possibilities.

To the extent we can clarify specific procedures, we are going to be successful in referring. People are wary of unlimited involvement in unknown relationships.

The actual introduction of the person needing help to the appropriate service may be done in one of two ways. Either one points the person to the service and lets him or her find the way, or one accompanies the individual and introduces him or her personally.

In a study of short-term cases in a family agency in New York City, L. S. Kegan distinguished between what he called "steering" and "referring" a client to another agency. He defined "referral" as a situation in which the caseworker takes the initiative to establish contact with the other resource on behalf of the client. In contrast, "steering" is a situation in which the client takes the initiative in contacting the other resource.

The results are striking. Eighty-two percent of those "referred" made contact with other resources, and of that group 74 percent were accepted for service. In contrast, only 37 percent of those who were "steered" made contact with other resources and of that group only 43 percent were accepted for service. Kegan concluded:

> That referral is generally more effective than steering in ensuring client contact with the other resource (and may possibly affect acceptance for service) seems clearly established by the reports from the other resources as well as the data obtained from the clients at follow-up.[20]

The optimum procedure for introducing the client to a service is to enable the person to take initiative for oneself. Whenever possible an individual is to be encouraged to take responsibility in contacting a service. Out of a mistaken understanding of what it is to help, the clergyperson often takes over for another. He or she is too eager to remove the obstacles, too eager for the individual to follow through on plans that have been worked out "for" the other. Practically, however, we may need to support the person through the referral contact more actively than we have thought.

At the steering end of the continuum (after the clarification process), the clergyperson may provide the individual with the name of the service, its telephone number, and its address. If the helper knows someone personally, he or she may say, "I suggest you call and talk with Mr. so-and-so. You may use my name if you care to." In effect, a letter of introduction has been given, but the individual must deliver it himself or herself.

At the other end of the continuum, the clergyperson takes the individual and introduces him or her directly to the helping service. That may be necessary with those who are immature, dependent, or ill. In some instances that may mean calling and arranging an appointment. In other instances it may even be necessary to arrange transportation to the service.

The extent to which the clergyperson takes initiative in establishing contact with a service on behalf of a parishioner ought to be arrived at by shared agreement. Once it has been established that the individual ought to be referred, and once it has been established to what service the individual is to be referred, then the actual mechanics can be decided upon jointly, even as intervention and interpretation were a matter of joint participation. The clergyperson may say something like this: "I'm not certain exactly how you would like to follow through on what we have discussed. There are a number of possibilities. I could give you the name, telephone number, and address of the agency and you could make your own arrangements. There would be no need to have me involved in the process. On the other hand, you might prefer to have me call and arrange an appointment for you and then let you know. Still another possibility would be for you to make your own appointment and let me know when it is going to be—then if you would like, I could call the worker and give her a little background on our relationship and the nature of your situation."

Regardless of how much or how little the clergyperson helps in the introducing process, the basic consideration is that the individual being referred participate in determining how the process will be carried out.

I began the discussion of referral by suggesting it is a way in which a person is referred by someone one trusts for purposes that one construes as being concerned with one's own welfare. The referral bridge consists of intervention, interpretation, and introduction.

In the end the helper is confronted with a paradox. On the one hand, one is asked to help and one knows that one can help. On the other, one realizes that one can only help in a preliminary and not an ultimate way. No individual, no matter how well trained or however wise, can know definitely and finally what is right for another human being. All genuine help must be based on humility:

> In the end you don't know what is right for another (you are lucky indeed if you know it for yourself); you don't have to face what he is facing (and pray God you never may have to); you don't, and never will, and pray God that you may never acquire that pride that dares to assert it does, or even some day may, know the length and breadth and the depth of a [person] . . . the more you know, the less you know or claim to know.[21]

Deep religious convictions ought to compel clergy to collaborate with other helping professionals. I believe that God is present in the world, not only in manifest and open form through the church, but also in latent and hidden form in human need. Wherever people struggle for justice, for order, for dignity, for well-being, God is present—incognito many times, but nevertheless there. Inasmuch as we respond to others in need, we are ministering unto Christ himself.

Biblically, we recognize the fact that people have differing gifts. The task of helping people be people, of humanizing humanity, of enabling every individual to find a place where he or she can consider himself or herself necessary within the whole of being[22] can be carried out and fulfilled by no single person or group. There are and have to be multiple ministries. The task of responding to human pain requires orchestration, not solo performances.

11

Too Much Sand: a changing strategy

"I have no time to bother about Joey and his problems."

One of my students had inquired about referral for Joey. Joey was a fourth grader the student had met through an assignment in an elementary school classroom. Plagued by multiple problems, Joey became the butt of his class's aggression. Joey's pain was acute, my student's intentions commendable, the referral question seemingly appropriate. My response sounded harsh, rejecting, unfeeling, insensitive. The student and his colleagues reacted with outrage to my apparent callousness.

"The world is full of Joeys," I began. Their reaction to this troubled child provided me with the opportunity to try to open up for them a re-viewing of what it might mean to respond. "You can spend all your time walking through the forest (of life) picking up twigs," I continued. "The woods are full of twigs. But the problem is the forest. If you spend much time picking up twigs, you will never get to the trees that produce the twigs."

Of course I was concerned with Joey—with all the Joeys—but in a way quite different from the student. In his view, Joey was the figure out in front—clear, focused, dominant   and the classroom was the ground—vague, diffused, secondary. By contrast, I perceived the classroom as the figure of explicit focus and Joey as the background of implicit concern. By that I mean a more viable way of responding to individual pain lies in dealing with the structures and systems in which people are embedded rather than in dealing with individuals in isolation. What at first sounded like a rejection of Joey came to be understood as an authentic caring for Joey. I was not as hardhearted as my students initially thought.

The press of societal problems in the 1960s—ranging from the quicksand war in Vietnam to urban riots to ecological disaster—has spread like cancer. No individual and no institution avoid the multiple diseases because we live in an interdependent world.

We also live in a pluralistic culture. Every individual and every institution participates in the world in a different way. These differences of perceived experience, understood events, and intended function must be taken into account in coping with the crises of our time.

In order for any institution to survive—on pragmatic grounds alone—it must be involved with the press of societal problems and with the viability of different approaches. Given our new interdependent world, every institution, including the church, is being required to re-view and redefine what it is about.[1]

The Problem

I have come to label this "re-viewing" of human pain as the problem of "too much sand and not enough mops." The image comes from an exchange between the Walrus and the Carpenter as they strolled along the beach in *Alice Through the Looking Glass:*

> "If seven maids with seven mops
> Swept it for half a year,
> Do you suppose," the Walrus said,
> "That they could get it clear?"
> "I doubt it," said the Carpenter,
> And shed a bitter tear."[2]

There was just too much sand and too few mops!

And that is what we are up against in the task of responding to human pain.

Too Much Sand

Consider the matter of too much sand.

Whether in churches or mental health centers or schools or

hospitals or agencies, people present themselves to the professional helper with clear and not so clear expressions of human pain. One observer has termed this group the "countable thousands" in contrast to the "hidden millions" who do not present themselves for help.[3] People who come seeking help make up only a tiny tip of the iceberg showing itself above the ocean of human suffering. Below the surface, out of sight—invisible to ordinary viewing—are the lonely, the lost, the unfeeling, the cut off, the crippled, the alienated. To revert to my basic image, there is simply too much sand—sand and sand and sand, everywhere—stretching on and on and on. . . .

In midtown Manhattan a few years ago, a research project assessed the mental health needs of an eight-block area. Prior to that time experts were estimating that between 12 and 15 percent of any adult population was in need of immediate professional services. The study disclosed that 80 percent of the adult population in that area could use immediate mental health service![4] A comparable study of a sparsely populated semi-urban and rural region a few years earlier had disclosed a similar picture. Only 15 to 20 percent of the populations studied were relatively free of crippling psychological difficulties.[5]

Startling!

When Erich Fromm wrote of "the sane society" twenty years ago, he was referring to our "insane" society. Time, tragedy, and turmoil have corroborated his point. What convention and culture have taken as sane has proven to be crazy; crazy in the sense that assumptions are unstable, reason is chaotic, emotions are eruptive, behavior is reactive, consequences are destructive. *Our whole society* is sick and desperately in need of healing. "Original sin" abounds!

Too much sand. . . .

Not Enough Mops

Even as needs are overwhelming, resources are inadequate. Conservative calculation suggests that "the *need* for mental health helping services outstrips formally measured *demand* by a factor of at least several hundred percent."[6]

We lack both maids and mops!

My own recital of the horrendous gap between available helping persons and anguished human pain would add little to existing documentation. Two colleagues in the field of community psychology, Melvin Zax and Emory Cowen, have reviewed and summarized in some detail several of the more pressing problems that confront the mental health field today. These include:

(1) substantial imbalances such that demand, and certainly need, for mental health services exceeds most categories of "supply" and resource;

(2) the acute and seemingly unresolvable shortages of professional manpower in all of the core mental health professions;

(3) the stubborn unwillingness of major classes of disorder, such as schizophrenia and the functional psychoses, to bend significantly to any of the multitude of solutions thus far developed;

(4) limits to the effectiveness, both clinically and socially, of principal techniques (such as psychotherapy) in the helping-kit of the mental health professional;

(5) the dramatic ineffectiveness, the limited reach, the questionable appropriateness of traditional mental health helping structures for vast segments of the population, which result in help being least available where it is most required.[7]

We do not even have nearly enough hospital beds, prison cells, probation offices, analysts' couches, therapists' chairs, clinic facilities to handle those hurting enough to mobilize themselves to seek help, let alone those hurting so badly and/or so unknowingly as to be unable to seek what limited help is available. While resources are being added, needs multiply geometrically.

Inadequate resources are shocking enough. The distribution of these resources, however, is even more disturbing.

Who gets the help that is available? Mostly those people and those areas that already possess a variety of resources: urban rather than rural; suburban rather than city; the gifted rather than the lacking; the winners rather than the losers; the ones that have rather than the ones that have not. With means go the means!

The people who are really helped tend to be all of a pattern. William Schofield in *Psychotherapy: The Purchase of Friendship* writes of the YAVIS syndrome in the helping professions. By this he means the kind of people we tend to respond to most often and most attentively: the young, the attractive, the verbal, the intelligent, the successful.[8] These are the ones we help, yet these are precisely the ones who have enough resources to make it somehow whether we specifically respond or not. In contrast, those who are old, unattractive, tongue-tied, unable to score well on standardized school exams, skilled with hands and feet instead of books and mouths—these are the people who tend not to be the recipients of helping attentiveness.

Perhaps Schofield exaggerates. Yet his perceptiveness penetrates existing cultural encapsulation. I must rely primarily on others for insight about the larger social scene of "principalities and powers."[9]

But on the more modest scale, the "principalities and powers" of mental health, I have developed expertise enabling me, even more, compelling me, to speak with some authority. While I have been politically alert through the years, I have also tended to be more spectator than participant. The larger problems loomed so large and my own resources looked so limited. In addition, early in my ministry my confrontation with acute human pain combined with my "natural" strengths in interpersonal relationships to focus my energies on more "therapeutic" endeavors. I devoted a large percentage of my time to working intimately with individuals. Gradually, that expanded to include working more intimately with groups. As a pastor, I always engaged in such work within the gestalt of the parish as background and the individuals and/or groups as the foreground. As a professor, I engaged in such work within the gestalt of the seminary as background and the individuals and/or groups as the foreground. However, in the last few years I have begun to wed my more personal therapeutic efforts with more structural political intention.

Perhaps "political" is too strong a word for what I am about. To me the term implies a larger focus on oppressive systems and structures that warp, misuse, abuse, and rape our humanity. That sounds more impressive than what in fact I am doing. Notwithstanding, to use the word "political" does suggest that I am construing my limited involvements as necessary and essential expressions of the larger task of liberation. I am finding that in many cases effective help for the individual can come only when the system of which the individual is a part can be changed.

Our understanding of abnormal psychology has undergone and is undergoing basic change. Problems have been increasingly defined in broader and broader ways: from the organic roots to intrapsychic dynamics to interpersonal interaction to systemic dysfunctioning, the scope of "abnormality" has grown. Whereas people previously saw only the disturbed individual, as in the encounter of Jesus with the demon-possessed man in Gerasenes, now we are seeing *the disturbing setting* in which such an individual lives and moves and has his or her being, namely, the marriage, the family, the neighborhood, the school, the organization, the community, the nation, the culture, the whole world.

With so much sand, no wonder there are too few mops and not enough maids.

Directions

Abraham Maslow once observed, "If the only tool you have is a hammer, you tend to treat everything as if it were a nail." [10]

Not dissimilarly, we in the helping professions have tended to view human crises primarily in individual terms. In some instances we have simply put on blinders, shutting out the larger context of pain and the deep sources of disruption. Much of the failure to cope effectively with these social and cultural crises must be attributed more to the nature of our institutions and approaches than to the attitudes and activities of isolated individuals. Intrapersonal and interpersonal strategies of social change tend to be both inadequate and inappropriate to deal with today's complexity. No longer can we responsibly minister to people one by one. Of necessity, we are driven to grapple with what Paul called "principalities and powers."

But how? That is the crucial issue.

Obviously, no single answer or any combination of answers will be "the" solution. Many answers and many approaches are called for—some having been tried are found fitting; others being tried end in uncertain consequences; still more are yet to be found and tried and altered in the light of experience. The day of the monolithic and the monopolistic in responding to human pain is long gone and best forgotten.

Regardless of particulars, the direction requires us to re-view—to see again and again and yet again—the dimensions of human pain. We are being compelled to expand our concern to reckoning with settings as well as selected individuals. We are being called upon to enlarge our goals to enhancing human potential as well as repairing human damage. In this time of transition we need different perceptual tools, more varied problem-solving skills, and a more inclusive vision of values.

In short, if we are to respond to full human hurt, we must see differently and act differently.

Different sights call forth differing tasks. What might some of those sights be? How might some of these tasks be carried out?

By looking at a concrete situation, I may be able to convey to you the substance of the re-viewing I am calling for. It is this situation in which sand and mops and maids became transformed for me from a confused and overwhelming muddy mess into a clearer and more manageable creative task.

It began quietly enough.

I had just finished speaking to an elementary school faculty about "schools without failure"[11] when the first question came: "What has been your experience with elementary school pupils?" I had had none, except for teaching a third- and fourth-grade church school class with my wife, plus having four children of our own.

Shortly afterward, a former teacher of one of our children came to tea. She gave the impression of being a strong and capable person. Karin, our daughter, had been in her class two years (second and third grades) and we were more than pleased with June's competence and creativity. After fourteen years she was a seasoned teacher.

With the tea, she started unburdening. Her classes had changed. This year she no longer felt sure. In fact, she was experiencing acute demoralization. In her class of twenty-six there were seven who exhibited clearly identifiable behavior problems calling for immediate professional help. There were boys throwing over desks and chairs, kicking and spitting and hitting. There was a girl who came in each day, pushed her desk back into a corner, stuck her thumb in her mouth and said nothing for the entire time. There was a brain-damaged boy who could only mumble unintelligibly. More than 30 percent of her pupils, and certainly she herself, were in need of direct attention.

Under the sand and mop and maid view I would have said, "June, maybe it would help if you were to get into therapy a couple of times a week or into a group to try to deal with your problems. Also you ought to refer those kids to the school mental health team for individual treatment."

Under a hammer approach, looking for nails to pound, I could have come up with seven youngsters for individual treatment, *if* the psychologist or social worker had any time in his or her one-day-a-week at that school, and June as a candidate for intensive psychotherapy at most or group therapy at least. The time invested in that classroom under the previous view could be close to ten to twelve hours per week for a long time. By seeing so much sand and so few mops and even fewer minds—deficits, pathology, problems, isolated individuals, sickness—the task would be too much, too trying, too impossible even to begin.

Fortunately, this was a period in my life when the re-viewing was coming. So I said to June, "You know, I have a problem as a result of my talk to that faculty. I need some experience with elementary school pupils. And you have a need. You need some help to cope with what is happening. Let me come into your classroom with you for the last twenty minutes of the day, for the next six weeks, and see what we can do."

Truly, we both believe—in retrospect—that God led us to each other.

In my re-view of that situation, I began seeing the classroom instead of individual pupils as the foreground. It was the pattern more than the parts. I began seeing human strength instead of damaging weaknesses as the foreground. It was the health of people more than the hurt that could emerge. I began seeing consultation instead of treatment service as the foreground. It was her job more than my job. I now saw delightful sand and a proper mop and an adequate maid instead of a muddy mess and a scarcity of mops and maids.

What was my new tool for this different task? How would we act differently now that we saw differently?

Following the approach of William Glasser, we proceeded to arrange the children in a circle (on their chairs in the middle of the room) for the last fifteen minutes of the day. The purpose: to talk together, to become more directly involved with each other as a group and as individuals, to listen to others as well as to speak oneself, to think critically, to make learning sensible by relating what was going on inside the classroom with what one was experiencing outside the school.

Teachers often tell me, "I always have discussions with my children. What is so different about what you are proposing?"

What I contend and what they fail to realize is that there are discussions and discussions. To sit in a circle is usually the first and basic difference. In the circle everyone is on the same level and everyone can see everyone else equally well. The built-in barriers of some being higher and others lower, or some taking in more and others taking in less, are eliminated. A second crucial difference lies in the rules or logic of the discussion. Most discussions are based on the premise that there are right and wrong answers: either what you say is true or it is false. Circle discussions are predicated on the assumption that there are no right or wrong answers.

In the circle one is freed from feeling foolish. This does not mean that one can be foolish or silly or dumb. Rather it means that one has one's own opinions, one's own hunches, one's own experience, one's own imagining. One can identify where one is without having to be somewhere else.

There are other rules for a circle meeting. Each of them is really a variation on the basic one of respecting each other and oneself. Children tend to elaborate on the rules, as people of all ages have developed commandments with their own supplementary commentary. "One person talks at a time." "We listen to each other." One kindergarten youngster came up with "Don't go to the bathroom in the circle meeting." He was getting the sense of attending to others at special times.

June and I started circle discussions with her class. To give her some idea of the process, I led the first few. Soon we were alternating regularly. I would take two a week; she three. This went on for six months and some ninety meetings.

At first the boy who had been throwing over desks and chairs continued to do so. We would have to pick him up (literally, at times) and remove him from the circle. Occasionally, he would stay outside the door until the meeting was over. Other times we would have to take him to the office. As the weeks passed, he stayed in the circle for longer periods. When he did act up, we would say, "That's it, Peter. You are saying you don't want to be in the circle today. You have to leave now. We will try again tomorrow."

In setting limits we were respecting the situation, ourselves, and Peter. He could not handle the demands of that moment. We were saying *he had made a choice*—by his behavior—as to what he wanted. We were following through in a logical and dependable manner on what was understood ahead of time: if you act up, you cannot remain in the circle. Peter, thus, could experience the consequences of his choices. Yet today's consequence never needed inevitably to be tomorrow's consequence. Each day was, in truth, a new day.

Gradually, Peter began to talk in the circle. He also began to listen. He had things he wanted to discuss. He had ideas he wanted to share.

The class talked about all kinds of things: monsters and motor cars, which little boys revel in; horses, with which little girls are fascinated. We also talked about problems: throwing spitballs, fighting, coming in late, talking after the bell rings, losing pencils, report cards.

Eddie kept losing his pencil. One day the class took that as "the class's" problem and not simply Eddie's.

"What is the problem?" I asked.

"Eddie keeps losing his pencil."

"It's not my fault," Eddie protested. "Others keep finding it and keeping it."

We were shifting from the isolated individual to a systemic interaction.

"Well, what can *we* do about it?" I responded. "You know, it's not just Eddie's problem. It's a problem for all of us."

"Tie a rubber band on the end of it."

"Take a piece of tape and write 'Eddie' on it. If anyone finds it on the floor, they can give it back."

"If we find any pencils on the floor, we can pick them up and put them right on the table nearest where we found them."

Such a process combines those two basic qualities of responding: namely, caring and cognitive development. The youngsters experienced themselves being attended to: they mattered, they were noticed, they were known. Equally, they found they were respected: their ideas, their needs, their experiences were taken seriously and thoughtfully.

As a teacher, June did not have time to give that kind of attention to twenty-six different children in isolation from each other. The presence of seven disrupting youngsters only compounded the predicament. Most of the day, teachers must teach subject matter, even though they try to respond to individual pupils. But in a circle, in ten minutes one can attend to twenty-six individuals in such a way that they each feel and know one's attentiveness. Out of doing that day after day, pupils come to know that the teacher knows they are there simply as themselves without demand, without evaluation, without qualification.

Motivation means involvement. As we become involved with each other and with tasks at hand, traction comes. Life moves with more satisfaction and more significance.

Glasser contends that the world can be divided into two groups: those who are making it and those who are not; the successes and the failures. Those who experience themselves as failures hesitate and resist involvement. If they let themselves be seen—by gesture or comment—they fear that even the right thoughts and the right deeds will somehow come out wrong for them.

But in the circle, even the most "wrong" comment comes out "right." In the circle there is no wrong way. In the circle there is just "your" way. Even more, in the circle one does not talk about what one does not know. No one feels much confidence in discussing ideas about which one is ignorant. Anyone can talk—and talk intelligently—about what he or she is interested in because one is an expert on that. One can talk about the chores one has to do at home because one is an expert on that. One can talk about what one likes to play because one is an expert on that. One knows one's own name better than anyone else. One can be secure in saying what one knows.

As one can say what one knows, one begins to experience a little more life space. And as one has more life space, one can allow others more life space. Collaboration replaces competition; inclusiveness takes over from exclusiveness. With more life space, each and all can begin to explore more of the unknown together and do it with excitement.

But involvement is never enough. In intense experiencing, the world can become irrational. We may be flooded by too many stimuli from outside as well as from inside. Then we are overwhelmed, unable to make sense of what we see and feel, incapable of acting on what we want and need. Catharsis has limited value. Getting feelings out is seldom enough. That may be only a first step in gathering up oneself, for contacting undifferentiated data activates primarily the right hemisphere—the receptive side. To own that experience and to utilize that data we equally need the left hemisphere—the active side.

Circle discussions emphasize critical thinking. They work on developing cognitive structure. Pupils are pressed to make discriminations and distinctions, to take stands on the basis of reasons and evidence, to figure out how to move into an unknown based on what one knows of a known.

One day Henry, the brightest youngster in the class, declared in a discussion on "superheroes" that "a superhero is one that can fly, that is strong, and does good."

The rest of the group went along with this definition, all, that is, except Jonathan, the brain-damaged boy. He leaned forward in his chair, his forearms resting on his thighs, his eyes intently centering on Henry across the circle, and reacted: "I disagree. Batman is a superhero and *he* doesn't fly."

Henry sat back in his chair, stunned. After a moment or two of reflecting, he replied, "You're right, I was wrong." What Henry meant was not that he-as-a-person was wrong, but that his thinking had not been critical enough so that his definition was inadequate.

Frustration with an immediate impasse need not be the end of a situation. Eddie, so often reduced to feelings of being "dumb" and "ugly," found that others had similar problems and that shared solutions could be found. Peter, so often exploding in impotent frustration and rage because of too heavy demands on his fragile ego structure, found he could gain recognition in ways that proved more satisfying both to himself and others. He also found that *he* had ideas that *he* wanted to talk about in the circle and that others were willing to talk about them with him. Quite unexpectedly, in the thirteenth week, June remarked spontaneously, "Why, Peter's thinking!"

Pupils learn that they can shape their world and not simply be molded by an environment. They can be active agents and not only receptive subjects. Beyond a minimum of factual information, what is really needed to make it in the world is a great capacity to imagine, to try out, to evaluate, to venture, to create, to collaborate. Problems confronting us are so complex that we need many vantage points and many alternatives and many values.

Schools Without Failure does not mean that no one ever experiences limits and limitations. That would be cause for despair. Rather, it means there is no point at which one finds oneself boxed in a corner without options. In educational jargon, it expresses the theological experiences of Exodus and Easter—liberation from whatever binds us to the past and terrifies us about the future.[12] Somehow resources can be rearranged to enable people to recover breathing space. There are other ways; there are unimagined-at-the-moment alternatives; there are untapped resources within people and in settings. There is a "beyond" in the midst of the "box," *if* we can see in other ways.[13]

The value of the circle discussion is seldom in any single meeting. Rarely does an issue or a problem or an idea stand out all by itself, unsupported by a gathering flow of events and experience. The cumulative effect of sitting down, eye to eye, on an equal basis, talking about things one is interested in, thinking about ideas that are intriguing, pays off. People become more genuinely who they truly are.

Significant involvement (being loved and loving) and satisfying behavior (self-respect and self-worth) transform human pain into human joy. That approach applies in the home and in an organization and in the community and around the world as well as in the classroom. It is adaptable to both a smaller setting and a larger realm.

I have tried to give you a glimpse of a sequence of events that served as a turning point in my understanding of the task confronting those of us who would respond to human pain. In that second-grade classroom, with a dedicated yet demoralized teacher and a group of ordinary and anxious youngsters, I discovered how too much sand and not enough maids and mops can be reconstrued in ways that make for life.

Based on that classroom and drawing upon similar experiences, let me set down explicitly what I regard as a different way to see and a different way to act in responding to human pain.

1. *We can see strength and not simply weakness.*

That means we emphasize the active quality of the left hemisphere, but in a way quite different from the exaggerated overintellectualization and overachievement drive that have so characterized it in the past. We work with the intentionality that is basic to every person.[14] To cope enhances one's ability to cope. There are dormant and hidden assets in every person and within each situation, needing only some kiss of awareness to be awakened and made known.

Even in our weaknesses, we are still strong (2 Corinthians 12:10).

2. *We can see people in process and not simply as finished products.*

Each experienced event both constitutes the effect of a configuration from the past and acts as a cause for further configuration in the future. Development and change are more fundamental than stasis and completion. Expectancy, the investing in and waiting upon that which lies ahead, influences the meaning and the management of every present. We have been imbued with "the breath of life" and thereby cannot *not* be active in "our" world.

Even in our arrivals, we are still on our way.

3. *We can see places of caring and not merely individuals needing care.*

The settings in which people interact are alive. They influence what does and does not happen. They predispose what can and cannot happen in those circumstances. To keep pupils at desks lined up in rows limits and allows quite different interaction than to place pupils in chairs in a circle. To deal with disturbed pupils and a disturbed teacher *in* the disturbing setting draws upon the intrapsychic dynamics of the separate individuals specifically in terms of their in-betweenness. There can be no escape from the constellation of forces precisely because we stay with that specific situation. Healing arises from within the system of interaction.

There are two corollary benefits to shifting the healing gestalt from figure to ground, from persons to places. The first is sheer *efficiency* in using available resources. Under the old view some ten to twelve hours per week of professional time were demanded, while under the new view at the very most (one half hour per day) only two and a half hours of professional time was expended. Under the old view the mental health professional was responsible for all the servicing, while under the new view the indigenous person (in this instance the teacher) was primarily responsible for servicing. The mental health professional acts primarily in the role of consultant. In geometric ratio, more people's needs are met by focusing on places of care than by preoccupation with individuals requiring care.

The second benefit is even more basic than efficiency, namely, *effectiveness*. The teacher's demoralization emerged primarily because of the exaggerated stress within the classroom. Of course, we could find etiological factors in her childhood, in her growing up, in her training, in her current life situation. Nevertheless, the classroom triggered the collapse, not some other factor. What went on between her and her pupils and among her pupils provided the material with which to work. There were all the ingredients. Within the actual interaction we have available the raw material out of which healthier patterns are built. The ways pupils responded were modified by the varied ways the teacher responded. Other means of satisfying needs for love and worth were discovered. The system that originally undermined now began to support and to strengthen. An accumulative effect converged. From having been dependent upon an outside savior, the peopled place became its own resource for healing. It generated its own potential health.

Even in dealing with individuals, we can focus on the places in which responding is called for.

4. *We can see regular routines of responding and not only emergency crises.*

Some needs are clearly developmental. They come at fairly predictable periods with rather typical features. We know they will be there and so we program for their arrival. Entrance into school (whether kindergarten, junior high, high, or college) activates anxiety in both students and parents. Activities of introduction that orient people to where they will be and what they will be doing and what they are likely to meet and how they might approach the demands all serve to lessen the stress of uncertainty, on the one hand, and to heighten the excitement of anticipation of the new, on the other.

The crises of the life cycle suggest one scaffolding from which to construct helping responses. The developmental needs of various age groups open a range of options for being with people where they are when they can optimally utilize human presence. Marriage groups focus on the development of intimacy. Liberation groups grapple with women's and men's liberation. Youth groups struggle with the formation of one's identity. There are groups for children and families and singles as well as groups for humanizing society. By getting people involved in their life experience intentionally and intelligently, we reduce the drain of their having to become involved resentfully and reactively as the result of unanticipated crises.

Timing constitutes a crucial variable in routines of responding. It includes not only the developmental clock, as I have just suggested, but also the circumstantial clocks. Special circumstances call for special caring. Where loss has come, we know that holidays, birthdays, and anniversaries all act to open the floodgates of grief. These are events in which the pain and the sadness again break into consciousness. These are moments when unfinished grief work can be continued most profitably. To be present to another in those times heals far more than to be around at other times.

Even in dealing with expected emergencies, we are not constricted to picking up the pieces in desperation. We are freer to work out more satisfying patterns with deliberation.

5. *We can cross systems for the "multiplier effect" and not stay within a single system with its incestuous consequences.*

I use the label "incestuous" deliberately. The sexual specter of inbreeding genetic weakness has its social specter. For like to stay with like only perpetuates selective inattention and behavioral limitation. Get any group of the same occupation together—clergy, psychologists, teachers, physicians, accountants, engineers—and the shared assumptions, the common experiences, the conventional conversations all serve to generate a single mind-set. Of course, any group is more varied than I have allowed in my caricature. My real point, though, is not about the individuals as individuals but about systems as systems. Because maintaining what exists consumes so much energy on the part of the participants, few, if any, systems can generate the extra energy necessary for significant system change. System incest tends to hinder innovative ideas and inspired action.

In April, 1972, Dennis Walsh became director of the Family Court of Monroe County (New York). Included in his revision of family probationary services was a group approach in contrast to the traditional individual approach both at the level of personnel and at the level of direct service. He was looking for some outside (the Court) leverage to move the system. I was looking for some outside (the seminary) linkage to educate students. Together we have developed and taught a seminar on "Small Group Theory and Practice." Half of the group have been probation officers from the court and half seminary students from the school. We have paired them as co-leaders responsible for conducting group treatment within the family court program. We have supervised them jointly as a group of co-leaders.

Two systems of authority (coercion and conscience) have crossed. Each has had to declare to the other what it is, how it operates, what it is about. Each has felt its limitations when exposed to the scrutiny of the other; also, each has experienced its unique assets as it works with the limitations of the other. Each has discovered it is more than it could be in and of and by itself. External persuasion requires internal considerations even as internal participation requires external considerations. Both tough realities and tender thoughtfulness are needed and both find reinforcement.

Seminary students could put more pressure on other probation officers to refer clients to the groups than could their probation officer colleagues. Too close association makes some kinds of confrontation more difficult. The presence of outside people quickens the activity of inside personnel.

Similarly, probation officers could confront seminary students with concrete human pain and complicated system problems more fully than ordinary classroom exercises could. Too much abstract discussion dulls and distorts the entangling web of structural maintenance and the unraveling fabric of personal needs. The immersion in real-world hurt sobers the romanticism of idea-world hopes.

The small input the seminarians have brought reinforces the yeast that is enriching the loaf of family court. The seminar is serving as stimulus and as modest resource for Walsh's re-vision.

Let me mention briefly two associated moves in the strategy of crossing systems. Circle discussion, reality therapy, and concern to connect one system with another converged with the introduction of Grand Rounds in Family Court. All court personnel—including judges—would gather to consider the many facets of a case or the many approaches to the need. For the first time every part of the system was present in one place with one focus: namely, to see and to share the intricate and subtle interdependency of Family Court.

For one program we brought a fifth-grade class to demonstrate group discussion techniques and to elaborate some of the principles as they might apply to Family Court. The presence of thirty excited youngsters transformed the staid and formal court into a charged and informal scene. The "audience" formed a large circle around the open space in the courtroom, made possible by removing the tables and chairs where lawyers and defendants usually sit. People were hanging over the judge's bench and out of the jury box and overflowing the visitor's section. The children and their teacher knelt or sat on the carpeted floor, very aware of the crowd yet very attentive to their task.

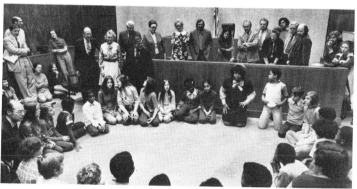

—Times-Union Photo—T. Gordon Massecar

A group of School 16 fifth graders and their teacher, Hannah Storrs, demonstrate group discussion techniques to Family Court judges and other court personnel. Nov. 16, 1972

"What is it like to be here in court?" the teacher, Hannah Storrs, asked them.

"Scary." "Strange." "Funny."

"Who are the judges and who are the criminals?" one youngster piped up.

"Can a woman be a judge?" wondered one of the girls.

And so the discussion moved.

Afterwards, Administrative Judge Robert Wagner took time to talk with them about the court. The staff had prepared doughnuts and juice, allowing twenty minutes for the operation. Of course, the children had gulped it all down in two minutes, leaving the staff taxed to the limit in handling the chaos. Some of the children admired the scarf and dress and shoes of an administrative secretary, telling her how lovely she looked and even hugging her. She, in turn, became so "high" from their presence that she hugged a judge and told him how great he was. And so the chain of contagion spread.

School children learned something about the Family Court system. Court personnel learned something about how courts were seen by children as well as what can happen when people are given the chance to talk together in a group in which there are no set answers. Both systems quickened with more life as a result of the crossing.

The next step in the multiplier effect was a joint Grand Rounds with the staff of the Rochester Community Mental Health Center. For several years the seminary has had students in training at the center. At that first conference the case of an adolescent arsonist was explored, drawing upon the demands of the court, the resources of the mental health system, and the front-line agonizing of the pastor related to the family. The limitations of each system—the court limited to coercion, the center limited to persuasion, the church limited to isolation—emerged more clearly. People fell between the cracks. People avoided help by pitting system against system. The desirability, even more the necessity, of the various systems collaborating as well as communicating stood out starkly.

One of the seminarians in the small-group course took initiative in arranging for a court group to meet at the center. Other liaison programs are developing between the two services. Mental Health Center staff are beginning to see clients at the court, and court personnel are spending time at the center. Through the model of co-leaders for groups, experienced group leaders are paired with less experienced group leaders to multiply the number of functioning group leaders. People from the court and the center and the church (mostly the seminary) are mixed together in co-leadership in both training and treatment.

In my enthusiasm for describing what is happening, I want to take care not to glamorize the results. While groups have taken root and blossomed in the center, they still struggle for existence in the court. While seminarians and clergy are involved, they are still supplementary and peripheral to the agencies. While more people are being touched, the ramifications of need continue to be horrendous.

In the model of crossing systems, inside power combines with outside impetus for more inspired implementation. People within one system (such as court or center) are stimulated and encouraged and enlarged and reconfirmed by their outside contacts. People outside that system but inside another (such as seminary or church) are stimulated and sobered and enlarged and reconfirmed by their inside contacts. Mutual learning occurs. Professional competence develops. Attentiveness to human pain grows. Unanticipated positive consequences appear.

Some retooling of responding skills is called for. Much ongoing support is essential. Intermittent reinforcement must occur. And out of the mix comes a little more healing, a bit more hoping, and a larger community of those who care. Even though we are rooted in a particular system, we give more and receive more than we ever imagined possible by virtue of crossing over the boundaries in collaborative responding.

One additional statement as to what I regard as a different way to see and a different way to act in responding to human hurt follows:
6. *We can act intentionally and not simply react spasmodically.*

To see and to act as I have been suggesting demands perspective and purpose and program. We need skills in analyzing social contexts in order to determine the issue of greatest concern to those who are part of that situation. Beyond that we need skills in assessing the relationship of various systems to those issues and then strategizing with and for those systems in terms of healing human pain.

In professional jargon, what I am alluding to carries the awesome label of strategic planning process. The basic elements of the model include identifying assumptions, agreeing upon objectives, arriving at strategies, and implementing tactics.

   a. A group clarifies the underlying premises upon which its purposes are based. In addition, the operational assumptions under which the system or institution is actually functioning are made explicit.
   b. The group states objectives that it wants to realize within a specified period of time. The objectives must be concrete enough so that actual progress can be determined.
   c. Once clear about objectives, the group explores multiple possibilities by which those goals can be reached. New ways of acting are stressed as the key in strategic planning.
   d. Finally, detailed steps are outlined as to who does what, when,

and where in order to complete the objectives.

Because of the intertwining of assumptions, objectives, strategies, and tactics, each of these areas is continually being revised in light of ongoing developments.

In order to have some flesh on these bare bones, let me describe one instance of its application.

The Council on Theological Education of the Board of Educational Ministries of the American Baptist Churches struggled for years with ongoing problems related to the preparation of professional leadership. Its influence was little, its expectancies less, its problems overwhelming. Dollars were scarce; demands were cancerous. At its annual meeting in 1972, the mushrooming cloud of institutional bankruptcy brought a tentative consensus that, unless the council acted in thoughtful and decisive ways, current frustration would turn into future futility. An overall plan for a nationwide strategy was called for.

But how to arrive at it and even more, to implement it if one could be developed?

I was invited to meet with the executive committee to undertake the task. We talked about their hopes. We looked briefly at their hurts. We dwelt at length on what they saw as obstacles. Next, a subgroup drew up a tentative plan. A second meeting (this time with additions to the group in order to begin the process of enlarging the circle of concern and commitment) re-viewed the purposes and revised the proposal. Having agreed upon what we were about, we proceeded to specify the steps needed to accomplish that:

—Who was important to have at the conference?
—Who would contact the names agreed upon in order to guarantee their participation?
—What background materials would be needed? When? Who would be responsible?
—How might a climate of awareness of the need and of anticipation of the agenda be created?

And so the glacier began to move. We were insuring results by carefully building in basic ingredients.

Let me make the process explicit: an initial *focus* of concern, an expanded *elaboration* of that concern, a tentative *refocusing* of the concern in terms of an implementing procedure, a further *expansion* by the inclusion of more concerns as additional people are drawn into the process, a *further focusing* of an agreed upon agenda that would lead to decisions and actions. There is an alternation between the larger group with its fuzzing phase and a subgroup with its focusing phase. With each refocusing there comes more clarity, more consensus, more commitment, more traction.

Without going into detail as to the working conference program, I want to lay out the general unfolding:

a. The general plan included:
   (1) Purpose
   (2) Objectives: identifying three crucial issues that each person individually was *wanting and willing to work on;* gathering specific ideas for action related to the issues; developing agreement and assigning responsibility for implementation.

b. The actual program process included:
   (1) *Orientation* to each other as persons and to background input.
   (2) *Issue development* in random groups to arrive at a consensus as to three crucial issues.
   (3) *Idea elaboration* to develop specific ideas for dealing with each of the issues. People worked in random groups, groups based on role responsibilities (e.g., administrators and faculty, national staff, trustees, etc.), groups based on geographical regions, and, finally, the conference group.
   (4) *Implementation strategy and tactics* through three task groups.

People had arrived at the conference with negative expectations and considerable resistance. Throughout the period they hung in despite defensiveness, uncertainty, and the demand for change. They left feeling less demoralized, more confident, and with specific steps to implement a denomination-wide strategy. From isolated, reactive, independent activity a more related, rational, collaborate understanding emerged.

Again, I would warn you not to assume that all problems were solved and all people satisfied. Yet more was accomplished than anyone imagined possible. The issue in the systems approach as much as in the individual approach is seldom the maximum distance covered and usually a minimum change in direction. As in sailing, at first the change seems so minute as to be insignificant. Over time those few degrees of difference stretch into significant directional consequences.

Even though we are constantly reacting to immediate and emergency situations, we take time to think through and plan strategically long-range responses to human pain.

Summary

Too much sand, not enough maids and mops—that was our presenting problem. By re-viewing and re-visioning what we see and what we do, we can transform an overwhelming task into a more manageable endeavor.

Previously, we concerned ourselves primarily with:

—pathology
—patients/individuals
—specialists
—rehabilitative treatment
—isolated people and situations
—spasmodic and emergency reactions.

Currently, we are also concerning ourselves with:

—potentialities
—community/systems
—everyone as participant/contributor
—preventive consultation
—inclusion of every related and relatable person and component
—intentional and planned action.

It would be illusory and utopian to act with the belief that through one's involvement all will work out well for everyone. The task of humanizing society is ongoing. No particular task matters ultimately; every particular task has a place in the swirling constellations of history. No one can do everything. Each one is called to do something.

A Jewish sage once observed, it is not incumbent upon us to finish the task, but neither are we free to desist.[15]

12

Risk

Responding . . .
> oneself as the key
> peace out of pieces and parts
> common features: relationship, place, rationale, procedures
> the whole person with bodily stress and two hemispheres of the
> brain
>
> confront us with the choice:
> ARE WE ABLE TO RESPOND?

Special pain . . .
> dependency with its masks of warmth and indifference and
> hostility
> aging with its poignancy of loss of mastery
> dying with its demand to humanize experience and determine
> meaning
>
> confront us with the truth:
> WE OURSELVES ARE

> DEPENDENT

> AGING

> DYING

A larger task . . .
> we need others to help our helping
> there are others

> too much need, too few resources
> a different task and different strategy
> systems and structures

> confront us with the demand:
> ## CHANGE OUR THINKING
> ## CHANGE OUR RESPONDING

In helping and being helped, we ordinarily begin and end with the individual, independent and isolated. The focus has applied equally to the helper and to the one helped. Always the split is between the self and the other, regardless of receiving or giving.

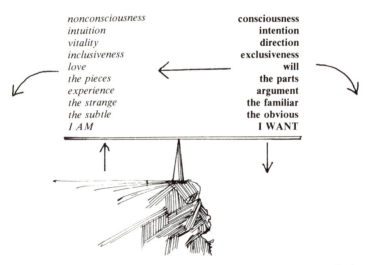

nonconsciousness	**consciousness**
intuition	**intention**
vitality	**direction**
inclusiveness	**exclusiveness**
love	**will**
the pieces	**the parts**
experience	**argument**
the strange	**the familiar**
the subtle	**the obvious**
I AM	**I WANT**

A Saul Steinberg cartoon dramatizes the split.[1] A seesaw balances on the edge of a precipice. Land stretches out to the left; space falls away on the right. A person stands upright at either end. The one in space holds a gun. It is aimed at the one over land. He fires the gun. A bullet pierces the air, heading straight for the heart of the other. The finale is clear: when the one over land falls off, the one in space hurtles down. There is no avoiding the inevitable. The loss of the victim means the demise of the victor.

The one in space represents all that we regard as solid, substantial, focused, clear, decisive. Here are clustered elements of the explicit expression "I want . . .": consciousness, intention, direction, will, the parts and the particulars of knowing by argument, the familiar and the obvious.

The one over land represents all that we regard as thin, superfluous, vague, diffused, indecisive. Here are clustered elements of the implicit expression "I am . . .": nonconsciousness, intuition, vitality, inclusiveness, love, the pieces and the patterning of knowing by experience, the strange and the subtle.

It does not matter what level of understanding we assume— biological, sociological, psychological, theological—the picture is clear. The part that we own—the consciously known—always balances over the precipice. The pieces that we do not possess—the intuitively sensed—always balance over land.

By destroying the balancing ends of the seesaw, we sabotage the whole. The clear part turns willful. It would exist without the other: intellect without intuition, content without context, communication without metacommunication, individual without relationship, people without structures. But only for a moment. Denial produces reversal. In taking over, the obvious is done in. In letting go, the subtle comes through.

Theologically, the precise form of the person/power in space is law—the systematic, the focused, the coherent ordering of life. The precarious presence of the person/power over land is gospel—the surprising, the spontaneous, the compelling bursting-out of living. In gestalt language, the flesh of the figure reflects the Word of the ground.

Under conditions of alienation, we have either too many parts and not enough pieces or too many pieces and not enough parts; exaggerated substance and no spirit or excessive spirit and no substance; will without love or love without will; judgment without mercy or mercy without judgment; individuals without community or community without individuals.

Under conditions of affirmation we have both parts and pieces, substance and spirit, power and meaning, freedom and destiny, persons and community, love and justice, me-with-you/you-with-me: together yet distinguishable.

. . . I and Thou, love and justice, dependence and freedom, the love of God and the fear of God, passion and direction, good and evil, unity and duality.[2]

"According to the logical conception of truth only one of two contraries can be true, but in the reality of life as one lives it they are inseparable. . . . The unity of the contraries is the mystery at the innermost core of the dialogue."[3]

The dialogue of life, as Martin Buber expressed it: within our own psyches, between each other, through the groups of which we are part, within community and throughout society.

Hope lies in discovering that the familiar here-and-now is always and ever present in the unfamiliar there-and-then, even as the unclear there-and-then is inevitably and necessarily present in the overly clear here-and-now.

In responding to human pain we risk what is known for what is yet to be known. We give up safety for searching. We lose life for the sake of life. If we are to respond, then we risk that risk.

To me, risking risk means trusting God!

In that trust I respond. . . .

References

Preface

[1] Jerome D. Frank, *Persuasion and Healing: A Comparative Study of Psychotherapy*, rev. ed. (Baltimore: The Johns Hopkins University Press, 1973), p. 15.

[2] Idries Shah, *The Sufis* (New York: Doubleday & Company, Inc., 1971), pp. 65-110.

[3] Idries Shah, *The Pleasantries of Mulla Nasrudin* (New York: E.P. Dutton & Co., Inc., 1971), p. 66.

Chapter ONE The Key

[1] Quoted in Shah, *The Sufis* (New York: Doubleday & Company, Inc., 1971), p. 232.

[2] Idries Shah, *The Pleasantries of Mulla Nasrudin* (New York: E.P. Dutton & Co., Inc., 1971), p. 82; Idries Shah, *The Sufis, op. cit.*, p. 91.

[3] Rollo May, *The Meaning of Anxiety* (New York: The Ronald Press Company, 1950), p. 48, footnote.

[4] Robert E. Ornstein, ed., *The Nature of Human Consciousness: A Book of Readings* (New York: The Viking Press, 1973), p. 166.

[5] *Ibid.*, pp. 436, 317.

[6] Rudolf Otto, *Mysticism East and West: A Comparative Analysis of the Nature of Mysticism*, trans. Bertha L. Bracey and Richenda C. Payne (New York: The Macmillan Company, 1960). pp. 29, 28.

[7] James B. Ashbrook, *The Old Me and A New i* (Valley Forge: Judson Press, 1974), pp. 87-91.

[8] Bernard Gunther, "Sensory Awareness and Relaxation." In Herbert Otto and John Mann, eds., *Ways of Growth* (New York: Grossman Publishers, 1968), pp. 60-68.

[9] James B. Ashbrook, "The Functional Meaning of the Soul in the Christian Tradition," *The Journal of Pastoral Care*, vol. 12 (Spring, 1958), pp. 1-16.

[10] *Realencyklopaedie fuer Protestantische Theologie und Kirche* (vol. 6, p. 453), quoted in Reinhold Niebuhr, *The Nature and Destiny of Man*, vol. 1 (New York: Charles Scribner's Sons, 1943), p. 151.

[11] Perry D. LeFevre, *The Prayers of Kierkegaard* (Chicago: University of Chicago Press, 1956), p. 36.

[12] Magda Proskauer, "Breathing Therapy," in Herbert Otto and John Mann, *op. cit.*, pp. 24-33.

[13] Frederick S. Perls, *Ego, Hunger and Aggression: The Beginning of Gestalt Therapy* (New York: Random House, Inc., 1969); Frederick S. Perls, Ralph F. Hefferline, and Paul Goodman, *Gestalt Therapy: Excitement and Growth in the Human Personality* (New York: Julian Press, Inc., 1951); Frederick S. Perls, *Gestalt Therapy Verbatim*, comp. and ed. John O. Stevens (Lafayette, Calif.: Real People's Press, 1969); Joen Fagan and Irma Lee Shepherd, eds., *Gestalt Therapy Now: Theory, Techniques, Applications* (New York: Harper & Row, Publishers, 1971); Erving and Miriam Polster, *Gestalt Therapy Integrated* (New York: Brunner/Mazel, Inc., 1973).

[14] Fagan and Shepherd, *op. cit.*, pp. 140-149.

[15] Paul Tillich, *The Eternal Now* (New York: Charles Scribner's Sons, 1963), pp. 26-35.

[16] Quoted in Otto, *op. cit.*, p. 80.

Chapter TWO A Case

[1] See footnote 13 in Chapter ONE, especially, Perls, *Gestalt Therapy Verbatim*, pp. 67-71; Perls, *Ego, Hunger and Aggression*, pp. 237-246; Perls, et al., *Gestalt Therapy*, pp. 211-224.

[2] I agreed to see her at the University of Rochester Counseling Center where the staff would observe us through a one-way mirror for teaching purposes. I am indebted to Dr. Forrest Vance, former director, and the staff for their support and encouragement. I am indebted even more to Rhonda (pseudonym) for sharing herself for the sake of others' growth as well as her own.

Chapter FOUR The Grammar

[1] Sören Kierkegaard, *The Concept of Dread*, trans. Walter Lowrie (Princeton: Princeton University Press, 1944), pp. 124-125.

[2] Hans H. Strupp, "On the Basic Ingredients of Psychotherapy," *Journal of Consulting and Clinical Psychology*, vol. 41 (August, 1973), pp. 7-8.

[3] Sol L. Garfield, "Basic Ingredients or Common Factors in Psychotherapy?" *Journal of Consulting and Clinical Psychology,* vol. 41 (August, 1973), p. 10.

[4] Jerome D. Frank, *Persuasion and Healing: A Comparative Study of Psychotherapy,* rev. ed. (Baltimore: Johns Hopkins University Press, 1973). See also Jerome D. Frank, "The Demoralized Mind," *Psychology Today* (April, 1973), pp. 22ff.

[5] Charles B. Truax and Robert R. Carkhuff, *Toward Effective Counseling and Psychotherapy: Training and Practice* (Chicago: Aldine-Atherton, Inc., 1967), pp. 23-143.

[6] Frank, *Persuasion and Healing, op. cit.,* p. 326.

[7] Mircea Eliade, *The Sacred and the Profane,* trans. Willard R. Trask (New York; Harcourt Brace Jovanovich, Inc., 1959), p. 28.

[8] Mircea Eliade, *Cosmos and History: The Myth of the Eternal Return,* trans. Willard R. Trask (New York: Harper & Row, Publishers, 1959), p. 17.

[9] *Ibid.,* pp. 12-21.

[10] Eliade, *The Sacred and the Profane, op. cit.,* p. 59.

[11] Morton A. Lieberman, Irvin D. Yalom, and Matthew B. Miles, *Encounter Groups: First Facts* (New York: Basic Books, Inc., Publishers, 1973), pp. 226-267; see also Morton A. Lieberman, "Behavior and Impact of Leaders," in Lawrence N. Solomon and Betty Berzon, eds., *New Perspectives on Encounter Groups* (San Francisco: Jossey-Bass, Inc., Publishers, 1972), pp. 135-170.

[12] Lieberman et al, *op. cit.,* pp. 434-435.

[13] Perry London, *The Modes and Morals of Psychotherapy* (New York: Holt, Rinehart and Winston, Inc., 1964), pp. 64-65.

[14] *Ibid.,* p. 116.

[15] *Ibid.,* p. 39.

Chapter FIVE The Whole Person

[1] Hans Selye, *The Stress of Life* (New York: McGraw-Hill Book Company, Inc., 1956), p. 255. Used with permission of McGraw-Hill Book Company.

[2] *Ibid.,* p. 32.

[3] *Ibid.,* p. 261.

[4] *Ibid.,* p. 11.

[5] *Ibid.,* p. 266.

[6] *Ibid.,* p. 267.

[7] *Ibid.,* p. 271.

[8] *Ibid.,* p. 31.

[9] Quoted in Idries Shah, *The Sufis* (New York: Doubleday & Company, Inc., 1971), p. xxvi.

[10] Robert E. Ornstein, *The Psychology of Consciousness: Readings from Scientific American* (New York: The Viking Press, 1973), pp. 50-51.

[11] *Ibid.,* pp. 49-73.

[12] *New York Times Magazine* (Sept. 9, 1973, Section 6).

13 Michael S. Gazzaniga, "The Split Brain in Man," in Robert E. Ornstein ed., *The Nature of Human Consciousness: A Book of Readings* (San Francisco: W. H. Freeman and Company Publishers, 1973), pp. 87-100; Ornstein, *The Psychology of Consciousness, op. cit.,* pp. 55-58.

14 Frederick Franck, *The Zen of Seeing: Seeing/Drawing as Meditation* (New York: Alfred A. Knopf, Inc., 1973), pp. 5-6. Used with permission of Alfred A. Knopf, Inc.

15 Lancelot W. Whyte, *Contemporary Psychology,* vol. 18 (July, 1973).

16 David Bakan, *The Duality of Human Existence* (Chicago: Rand McNally & Company, 1966), p. 15.

17 *Meister Eckhart, a Modern Translation,* trans. Raymond Bernard Blakney (New York: Harper & Row, Publishers, Harper Torchbooks, 1941), p. 232.

Chapter SIX The Guts

1 Robert Bretall, ed., *A Kierkegaard Anthology* (Princeton: Princeton University Press, 1951), p. 19.

2 Alan Keith-Lucas, "The Nature of the Healing Process," *The Christian Scholar,* vol. 43 (Summer, 1960), pp. 119-127. See also Alan Keith-Lucas, *Giving and Taking Help* (Chapel Hill: University of North Carolina Press, 1972). The basic points in this chapter have been adapted and altered from James B. Ashbrook, *In Human Presence—Hope* (Valley Forge: Judson Press, 1971), pp. 87-102.

3 Keith-Lucas, *Giving and Taking Help, op. cit.,* p. 48.

4 Susan C. Anderson, "Effects of Confrontation by High- and Low-Functioning Therapists," *Journal of Counseling Psychology,* vol. 15 (1968), p. 411.

5 *Ibid.,* p. 413.

6 Carl R. Rogers, *On Becoming a Person* (Boston: Houghton Mifflin Company, 1961), p. 52.

7 Cited by John Hutchinson, *Faith, Reason and Existence* (New York: Oxford University Press, Inc., 1956), p. 84.

8 Keith-Lucas, *Giving and Taking Help, op. cit.,* p. 53.

9 Eugen Rosenstock-Huessy, *The Christian Future or The Modern Mind Outrun* (New York: Charles Scribner's Sons, 1946), pp. 116-117.

10 Keith-Lucas, *Giving and Taking Help, op. cit.,* p. 117.

11 Morton A. Lieberman, Irvin D. Yalom, and Matthew B. Miles, *Encounter Groups: First Facts* (New York: Basic Books, Inc., Publishers, 1973), p. 441.

12 Walter Lowrie, *A Short Life of Kierkegaard* (Princeton: Princeton University Press, 1942), p. 160.

Chapter SEVEN Dependency

1 Victor White, *Soul and Psyche* (New York: Harper & Row, Publishers, 1960), p. 173.

2 My initial venture in developing such a cognitive map appeared in *In Human Presence—Hope* (Valley Forge: Judson Press, 1971), pp. 185-212.

That material, while still basic, came through as too technical and too complicated to understand and utilize easily. I enlarged the map from the interpersonal level to the cosmological level in *Humanitas: Human Becoming and Being Human* (Nashville: Abingdon Press, 1973), pp. 117-137. For those wanting to delve more deeply into the theoretical background see Timothy Leary, *Interpersonal Diagnosis of Personality* (New York: The Ronald Press Company, 1957) and Robert C. Carson, *Interaction Concepts of Personality* (Chicago: Aldine-Atherton, Inc., 1969).

[3] Roger John Williams, *You Are Extraordinary* (New York: Random House, Inc., 1967).

[4] Frederick S. Perls, *Gestalt Therapy Verbatim,* comp. and ed. John O. Stevens (Lafayette, Calif.: Real People Press, 1969), pp. 17-19.

[5] Leary, *op. cit.,* p. 65, labeled these patterns: the docility of the dependent personality, the masochism of the self-effacing personality, and the rebelliousness of the distrustful personality. Everett L. Shostrom, *Man, the Manipulator* (Nashville: Abingdon Press, 1967), pp. 36-38 called them: the clinging vine, the weakling, and the judge. I draw upon Karen Horney, *The Neurotic Personality of Our Time* (New York: W. W. Norton & Company, Inc., 1964) for understanding neurotic claims, the tyranny of the should, self-hate and self-contempt, the appeal of love by the self-effacing, morbid dependency, and the appeal of freedom by those who are resigned.

[6] Horney, *op. cit.,* p. 110.

[7] Idries Shah, *The Sufis* (New York: Doubleday & Company, Inc., 1971), p. 66.

Chapter EIGHT Aging

[1] Simone de Beauvoir, *The Coming of Age,* trans. Patrick O'Brian (New York: G. P. Putnam's Sons, 1972), p. 2.

[2] *Ibid.,* p. 283.

[3] Idries Shah, *Caravan of Dreams* (London: The Octagon Press, 1968), p. 155.

[4] Clark Tibbits, ed., *Handbook of Social Gerontology* (Chicago: University of Chicago Press, 1960), pp. 9-10.

[5] Wilma Donahue, "Rehabilitation of Long-Term Aged Patients," in Richard H. Williams, Clark Tibbits, Wilma Donahue, eds., *Processes of Aging: Social and Psychological Perspectives,* vol. 1 (New York: Aldine-Atherton, Inc., 1963), p. 541.

[6] Robert J. Havighurst, B. L. Neugarten, and S. S. Tobin, "Disengagement and Patterns of Aging," in Bernice L. Neugarten, ed., *Middle Age and Aging: A Reader in Social Psychology* (Chicago: University of Chicago Press, 1968), pp. 161-172.

[7] Bernice L. Neugarten, Robert J. Havighurst, and Sheldon S. Tobin, "Personality and Patterns of Aging," in Neugarten, *op. cit.,* pp. 174-177. The information following is from this study.

[8] Margaret Kuhn, "The Gray Panthers," *Parade/The Sunday Bulletin* (Philadelphia, January 28, 1973).

[9] James C. Folsom, "Reality Orientation for the Elderly Mental Patient," *Journal of Geriatric Psychiatry,* vol. 1 (Spring, 1968), pp. 291-307; "Treatment Team, Tuscaloosa Veterans Administration Hospital, Attitude Therapy and the Team Approach," *Mental Hospitals* (November, 1965), pp. 307-320. I am indebted to St. Ann's Home for the Elderly, Rochester, New York, and specifically to Paul Duffy, M.D., and Mrs. Jean Donato, RN, for introducing me to Reality Orientation and Attitude Therapy.

[10] Erik H. Erikson, *Identity and the Life Cycle: Selected Papers* (New York: International Universities Press, 1959), p. 102.

[11] *Ibid.,* p. 98.

[12] Richard H. Williams, "Changing Status, Roles, Relationships," in Williams et al, *op. cit.,* pp. 261-297.

[13] Margaret E. Kuhn, "The Church in Ministry with Older Adults," Thesis Theological Cassettes, vol. 4, no. 6 (1973).

Chapter NINE Dying

[1] Idries Shah, *The Exploits of the Incomparable Mulla Nasrudin* (New York: Simon and Schuster, 1966), p. 119. Reprinted by permission of Collins-Knowlton-Wing, Inc. Copyright © 1966 Mulla Nasrudin Enterprises Ltd.

[2] See Michael G. Michaelson, "Death as a friendly onion," *New York Times Book Review* (July 21, 1974), pp. 6-8, for a perceptive review of the literature on the subject in the last twenty years.

[3] Herman Feifel, ed., *The Meaning of Death* (New York: McGraw-Hill Book Company, 1959); Bernard Spilka in "Death and Cultural Values: A Theory and a Research Program" (mimeographed paper presented at the American Psychological Association Convention, 1967) expanded the perspectives in Feifel into a theory of attitudes toward death and developed empirical scales to ascertain their relationship with other variables.

[4] Margaretta K. Bowers, Edgar N. Jackson, James A. Knight, Lawrence LeShan, *Counseling the Dying* (New York: Thomas Nelson Inc., 1964), pp. 6-7.

[5] E. G. LaForet, "The 'Hopeless' Case," *Arch. Internal Medicine,* vol. 112 (September, 1963), pp. 68-80; "Physicians Urged to Tell the Dying," *New York Times* (Jan. 9, 1966), p. 1.

[6] LaForet, *op. cit.*

[7] Hattie R. Rosenthal, "Psychotherapy for the Dying," *Pastoral Psychology* (June, 1963), p. 52.

[8] *Ibid.*

[9] Elisabeth Kübler-Ross, *On Death and Dying* (New York: The Macmillan Company, 1969).

[10] Sidney Jourard, *The Transparent Self* (New York: Van Nostrand Reinhold Company, 1964).

[11] Kübler-Ross, *op. cit.,* pp. 28-37.

[12] *Ibid.,* pp. 42-45.

[13] Sam Banks, "Dialogue on Death: Freudian and Christian Views" *Pastoral Psychology* (June, 1963), p. 47.

Chapter TEN The Use of Others

[1] Jean Paul Sarte, *No Exit and The Flies,* 10th printing (New York: Alfred A. Knopf, Inc., 1967), p. 38. Used with permission of Alfred A. Knopf, Inc.

[2] Gerald Gurin, Joseph Vernoff, and Sheila Feld, *Americans View Their Mental Health: A Nationwide Interview Survey* (New York: Basic Books, Inc., Publishers, 1960).

[3] Richard V. McCann, *The Churches and Mental Health* (New York: Basic Books, Inc., Publishers, 1962), p. 69.

[4] Joint Commission on Mental Illness and Health, *Action for Mental Health* (New York: Basic Books, Inc., 1961), pp. 104, 136.

[5] Harold Twiss of Judson Press has called to my attention a book being published at the same time as this one, *Comprehensive Pastoral Care* by Samuel Southard (Valley Forge: Judson Press, 1975), which describes how clergypersons may work with others to meet human need.

[6] McCann, *op. cit.,* p. 195.

[7] Grace C. Mayberg, "The Caseworker: Key to Building the Agency's Reputation," *Social Casework,* vol. 42 (November, 1961), pp. 451-456.

[8] Arnold Purdie, "The Minister and Community Services," *Pastoral Psychology,* vol. 10 (June, 1959), pp. 9-17.

[9] Grace C. Mayberg, *op. cit.,* p. 456.

[10] Helen E. Terkelson, *Counseling the Unwed Mother,* 2nd printing (Philadelphia: Fortress Press, 1970).

[11] Wayne E. Oates, *The Christian Pastor* (Philadelphia: The Westminster Press, 1964), pp. 220-236.

[12] Jules V. Coleman et al, "A Comparative Study of a Psychiatric Clinic and a Family Agency: Part II," *Social Casework,* vol. 38 (February, 1957), p. 79.

[13] Alan Keith-Lucas, "The Nature of the Helping Process," *The Christian Scholar* (Summer, 1960), p. 127. The following information is taken from this article.

[14] *Ibid.,* p. 121.

[15] Mary C. Anderson et al, "The Content of First-Year Field Work in a Casework Setting: Part II," *Social Casework,* vol. 34 (March, 1953), p. 113.

[16] Leona E. Tyler, *The Work of the Counselor,* 2nd ed. (New York: Appleton-Century-Crofts, 1961).

[17] Lawrence M. Brammer and Everett L. Shostrom, *Therapeutic Psychology: Fundamentals of Counseling and Psychotherapy,* 2nd ed. (Englewood Cliffs, N.J.: Prentice-Hall, Inc., 1968), p. 124.

[18] Celia Benney, "The Role of the Caseworker in Rehabilitation," *Social Casework,* vol. 36 (March, 1955), p. 121.

[19] Delwin M. Anderson and Frank Kiesler, "Helping Toward Help: The Intake Interview," *Social Casework,* vol. 35 (February, 1954), p. 72.

[20] Leonard S. Kegan, "The Short-Term Case in a Family Agency, Part II. Results of Study," *Social Casework,* vol. 38 (June, 1957), p. 301.

[21] Keith-Lucas, *op. cit.,* p. 126.

[22] Paul Tillich, "The Philosophy of Social Work," *Pastoral Psychology* (December, 1963), p. 27.

Chapter ELEVEN Too Much Sand

[1] James B. Ashbrook, "No Longer One by One: Ministry to Structures," in G. Douglass Lewis, ed., *Explorations in Ministry* (New York: IDOC Dossier, 1971), pp. 14-26. I am indebted to Kenneth Dean, Larry Coppard, and Ronald Richardson for educating me in some of the implications of structures, systems, and the political focus in response to human pain. I am even more in debt to H. Rhea Gray, executive director, and the W. Clement and Jessie V. Stone Foundation for grants enabling me to experiment in these areas.

[2] Lewis Carroll, *Alice in Wonderland*, authoritative texts, ed. Donald J. Gray (New York: W. W. Norton & Company, Inc., 1971), p. 141.

[3] William Schofield, *Psychotherapy: The Purchase of Friendship* (Englewood Cliffs, N.J.: Prentice-Hall, Inc., 1964).

[4] Leo Srole, Thomas S. Langner, Stanley T. Michael, Marvin K. Opler, and Thomas A. C. Rennie, *Mental Health in the Metropolis*, vol. 1 (New York: McGraw-Hill Book Company, Inc., 1962).

[5] Dorothea C. Leighton, "The Distribution of Psychiatric Symptoms in a Small Town," *American Journal of Psychiatry*, vol. 112 (March, 1956), pp. 716-723.

[6] Melvin Zax and Emory L. Cowen, *Abnormal Psychology: Changing Conceptions* (New York: Holt, Rinehart and Winston, Inc., 1972), p. 386.

[7] *Ibid.*, p. 403.

[8] Schofield, *op. cit.*, p. 133.

[9] A sample of my "mighty cloud of witnesses" to our sin-sick society includes the following: Franz Fanon (in *The Wretched of the Earth*) lays bare the violence to the human spirit of racism and colonialism. Thomas Szasz (in *The Manufacture of Madness* and *The Myth of Mental Illness*) alerts us to sinister social bondage of "an excessively psychiatrized society." R. D. Laing (in *The Politics of Experience*) attempts to document our contemporary violation of other selves and our experience. Paulo Freire (in *Pedagogy of the Oppressed*) develops an educational strategy to take action against the oppressive elements of "reality." James Cone (in *A Black Theology of Liberation*) contends that Christianity is a religion of liberation for the oppressed, especially blacks. Harvey Cox (in *The Seduction of the Spirit*) exposes the abuse of people's religion in the vast combination of technology, propaganda, exploitation, and imperialism that shut out the light of life as he witnesses to the use of the religions of the losers for the humanization of human beings.

[10] Quoted in Robert E. Ornstein, ed., *The Nature of Human Consciousness: A Book of Readings* (San Francisco: W. H. Freeman and Company Publishers, 1973), p. 3.

[11] William Glasser, *Schools Without Failure* (New York: Harper & Row, Publishers, 1969). I am indebted to June Chisholm for "baptizing" me into the world of elementary education and also to Glasser and the staff of his Educator Training Center for encouraging my work in this area.

[12] Harvey Cox, *The Seduction of the Spirit: The Use and Misuse of People's Religion* (New York: Simon and Schuster, 1973), pp. 152-153.

[13] James B. Ashbrook, *be/come Community* (Valley Forge: Judson Press, 1971), pp. 21-34.

[14] The gestalt clues discussed in the first chapter are suggestive of a means of building up one's will. See also Roberto Assagioli, *Psychosynthesis: A Manual of Principles and Techniques* (New York: Hobbs, Dorman & Co., Inc., 1969).

[15] Quoted in Erich Fromm, *You Shall Be as Gods* (New York: Holt, Rinehart and Winston, 1966), p. 157.

Chapter TWELVE Risk

[1] Paul Tillich, *My Search for Absolutes* (New York: Simon and Schuster, with drawings by Saul Steinberg, 1967), p. 114.

[2] Maurice S. Friedman, *Martin Buber: The Life of Dialogue* (Chicago: University of Chicago Press, 1955), p. 3.

[3] *Ibid.,* quoting Martin Buber, *Israel and the World, Essays in a Time of Crisis* (New York: Schocken Books Inc., 1948), "The Faith of Judaism," p. 17.

Index